Missing Persons

Auto/biography is currently one of the most popular literary genres, widely supposed to illuminate the study of the individual and his or her personal circumstances. *Missing Persons* suggests that auto/biography is, in fact, based on fictions, both about the person and about what it is possible to know about any one individual.

Organised into chapters which consider particular kinds of auto/biographical writing, such as work on the British Royal Family and auto/biographies of twentieth-century men, this book demonstrates the absences and evasions – indeed the 'missing persons' – of auto/biography. It will provide invaluable reading for students of women's studies, sociology and cultural studies courses.

Mary Evans is Professor of Women's Studies and Head of the Department of Sociology, University of Kent at Canterbury.

Missing Persons

The impossibility of auto/biography

Mary Evans

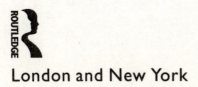

London and New York

First published 1999
by Routledge
11 New Fetter Lane, London EC4P 4EE

Simultaneously published in the USA and Canada
by Routledge
29 West 35th Street, New York, NY 10001

© 1999 Mary Evans

Typeset in Baskerville by Refinecatch Limited, Bungay, Suffolk
Printed and bound in Great Britain by
Clays Ltd, St Ives PLC

British Library Cataloguing in Publication Data
A catalogue record for this book is available from the British Library

Library of Congress Cataloging in Publication Data
Evans, Mary
  Missing persons : the impossibility of auto/biography / Mary Evans.
      p.   cm.
  Includes bibliographical references and index.
  1. Biography as a literary form. 2. Autobiography. I. Title.
CT21.E83 1999
808'.06692–dc21   98–19232
                                                                        CIP

ISBN 0–415–09975–7 (hbk)
ISBN 0–415–09976–5 (pbk)

Contents

Acknowledgements

Many people have helped me in the production of this book. In order to try to prevent them becoming 'missing persons', I should like to thank them here for their support and assistance. Sue Sherwood, Sally Wilcock and Sally Harris have given endless help to an author who finds it impossible to write with anything except a pen. I am deeply grateful to all of them for their grace and patience. Michael Bird read the completed manuscript with great care; I am indebted to him for his careful and helpful work. In its early stages this project was supported by a grant from the Nuffield Foundation, and I would like to thank them for their assistance.

I have presented parts of this book as papers at the universities of Sussex, Lancaster, Warwick, Manchester and the London School of Economics. I would like to thank all those institutions for their hospitality, and Celia Lury, Liz Stanley, Beverley Skeggs, Henrietta Moore and Alan Sheridan for their invitations to speak. Many people have listened patiently while I have talked about auto/biography; many others have contributed information about their own biographies and those of others. So my thanks are due to Anne Seller, Ros Coward, Janet Sayers, Jan Montefiore, Pat Macpherson, Audrey Lane and Barbara Einhorn for their understanding conversations. David, Tom and Jamie Morgan have unfailingly demonstrated the rich and rewarding diversity of human existence.

Every effort has been made to obtain permission to quote from the copyright works reproduced. In particular, the publishers would like to thank the following for their permission to include material in this book:

The Mandarins by Simone De Beauvoir. Reproduced by permission of HarperCollins Publishers Ltd.

Down and Out in Paris and London by George Orwell, Copyright © George Orwell 1933 and *The Road to Wigan Pier* by George Orwell, Copyright © George Orwell 1937. Reproduced by permission of Mark Hamilton as the Literary Executor of the Estate of the Late Sonia Brownell Orwell and Martin Secker & Warburg Ltd.

Brideshead Revisited by Evelyn Waugh. Reproduced by permission of the Peters Fraser & Dunlop Group Ltd.

The Protestant Ethic and the Spirit of Capitalism by Max Weber, 1958. Reproduced by permission of Prentice Hall.

French Lessons by Alice Kaplan, Copyright © Alice Kaplan, 1994. Reproduced by permission of the University of Chicago Press.

How Far Can You Go? by David Lodge. Reproduced by permission of Secker & Warburg Ltd (part of Random House UK).

The Auto/biographical I by Liz Stanley, 1992. Reproduced by permission of Manchester University Press, Manchester, UK.

Chapter 1

The possibilities of auto/ biography

Anyone who visits a public library or a bookshop in Britain will know that auto/biography is a flourishing literary genre. The shelves are packed with accounts of the lives of the great, the good, the bad and – increasingly as the democratisation of the genre has taken hold – the socially insignificant and powerless. The kings and queens are there, as are the politicians and the statesmen, but so too are the 'ordinary people'. This book is thus not about a process of literary or social exclusion – its thesis is not that these 'ordinary' people, the Mrs and Mr Jones of social life, have been left out by biographers. The Joneses do not (yet) have as much space as the Mountbattens and the Macmillans of this world, but they are there. The thesis in not, therefore, about who is left out, but about the ways in which the genres of auto-biography and biography cannot represent what they claim to represent, namely the 'whole' life of a person. Furthermore, this 'whole' person is in any case a fiction, a belief created by the very form of auto/biography itself. We are accustomed to classify autobiography as non-fiction, and yet it may be useful to think of it not as such, but as a mythical construct of our society and our social needs. Central to those social needs is the compelling wish of many people to experience life as an organised and coherent process, in which rational choices are made. Critics of twentieth-century society, from Freud and Weber to Kristeva and Gillian Rose, have all observed that the fear of inner, individual chaos is all too frequently projected on to the world as a desire for social order.[1]

The conventional expectation about auto/biography is, of course, that in the process of documenting an individual's life, something approaching the truth about that individual will be told. The 'need to know' is a priority in the telling of tales about individuals, and that endless fascination which we all have with the lives of others. From this viewpoint, it is obviously possible to see auto/biography as the literary equivalent of gossip. Instead of the verbal exchange of information about others which is a general social characteristic, the authors of autobiography use print to record and document individual lives. The difference, of course, is that we tend to view gossip as in some sense partial, while auto/biography is generally assumed at least to aspire to some version of absolute and inclusive truth.

If this is one of the general assumptions about auto/biography, then there are also others which characteristically inform writing about the genre. The first of these assumptions is that auto/biography is as old as literacy itself. Although it has now become conventional to distinguish between 'modern' and 'pre-modern' biography, there are assumed similarities in the form which stretch from Plutarch to the latest book on Princess Diana. Plutarch's *Lives* belongs emphatically to the pre-modern; even by the standards of the contemporary rearrangement of time and chronology, it is difficult to situate a book written in the first century AD as anything other than pre-modern. But the exact point of the separation between modern and pre-modern remains contentious. In his biography of King Alfred the Great, published in 1995, Alfred Smyth argues that:

> Asser's *Life* of King Alfred occupies a central place in Eng-
> lish historical writing, not only because of its acceptance by
> scholars as the earliest extant biography of an English king –
> and indeed of any English lay person – but because its sub-
> ject is Alfred the Great of Wessex whom Asser, the author of
> the *Life*, claims to have known as a tutor and a friend. The

immediacy of this extraordinary source is heightened by the author's claim to be writing his biography while the king was still living – in Alfred's forty-fifth year – in AD 893.[2]

Thus we have here the placing of the 'first' English biography in the ninth century AD – later than Plutarch but rather earlier than some of the other commonly aired 'first' biographies, such as Boswell's *Life of Johnson* or Froude's *Carlyle*. But what is striking about this potential 'first' in biography is that the ninth-century biographer is, as Smyth points out, obsessed with Alfred's relationship to literacy. 'He [Alfred] is obsessed with his own personal need to overcome illiteracy' writes Alfred's twentieth-century biographer. Thus we have a relationship which spans over a thousand years of history: a desire on the part of individuals to write and to record both their own histories and the histories of other individuals. Alfred the Great could not tolerate his own illiteracy, and in this lies an essential ingredient of auto-biography: individual terror at the thought of dying without a written record. In the latter part of the twentieth century, people living in industrial society take for granted written records about themselves: we acquire a personal biography whether we like it or not. For many millions of people living outside the societies of generalised literacy and bureaucratic documentation, this is not the case, and so autobiography has to be located as a literary genre that is an important part, not of culture generally but of literate cultures which are motivated by a desire to record.

While literacy and auto/biography go hand in hand, this cannot obscure the sense in which other cultures (and indeed our own) depend heavily on mythologised accounts of individual lives for the transmission of moral and cultural values. Nursery rhymes and fairy-tales in Western cultures are organised around individuals, and their part in organising auto/biography is an important one to which this account will return later. Those moral tales which children are told, or learn, about the greedy child, or the boy who cries 'Wolf, wolf', are all part of the cultural values which inform the more sophisticated form of autobiography. Indeed, throughout the nineteenth and twentieth centuries there has been a steady production of autobiographies and biographies which are organised as moral tales: overcoming specific hardships or illnesses, living through difficult times or finding personal happiness all have much in common with the narrative of Grimms' *Fairy Tales* or Bunyan's *Pilgrim's Progress*. What is striking about many of these tales is that the language of Bunyan becomes the language of the contemporary tale of battles against drug abuse or eating disorders: 'I picked up the burden of my problems' is a sentence which can be replicated over and over again in this literature.

But the autobiographies that fill the shelves of public libraries and are bought in large numbers by the reading public are not, on the whole, the explicitly moral tales about victories over illness or adversity, they are the scholarly accounts of individual lives which are given serious attention in the academic press and in critical circles. There are, in this exercise in recognition, 'serious' and 'good' auto/biographies which are reviewed with lengthy and careful attention, and which give rise to complex debates about the limits, the meaning and the responsibilities of the auto/ biographer. As such, auto/biography has the same intellectual status as the novel or poetry, it is a recognisable genre and one worthy of critical attention. As anyone who has visited a book- shop must know, there is an enormous amount of auto/ biography which is both trivial and superficial, but in the main the form (like the novel and poetry) has held its boundaries and can be recognised as a particular literary form. Indeed, in the past forty years, auto/biography has enjoyed a particular popu- larity as a result of two shifts in the practices surrounding litera- ture. The first is that auto/biography is now allowed (indeed expected) to reveal everything that can be found about an indi- vidual. While it was once the case that biographers were expected to draw veils of secrecy and evasion over particular matters (largely sexual ones), it is now the case that no matter in an individual life cannot, indeed should not, be revealed.

The work which was responsible for doing much to shift the

boundaries of revelation was Michael Holroyd's biography of Lytton Strachey, which was published in 1967.[3] Holroyd was not the first person – by far – to write about Strachey and the Bloomsbury group, but he was the first to provide comprehensive and explicit information about the sexual practices and choices of this most influential group of friends and relations. The comments by D.H. Lawrence, and later George Orwell, about 'the buggers' of Bloomsbury had revealed to anyone who was interested the sexual orientation of members of the charmed circle, but these kinds of throw-away comments (even though they were accompanied in the case of Lawrence and Orwell by a deep distrust of 'the buggers' and their work) were not the same as the documented and careful evidence collected by Holroyd about the complicated pattern of friendships within the Bloomsbury group. The individual most explicitly protected by previous biographers had been John Maynard Keynes. A life of Keynes by Roy Harrod (published in 1951) had made no mention of Keynes's homosexual relationships (in particular with Duncan Grant) but had used the commonplace euphemism of 'friend' to describe the affairs that Keynes had with men prior to his marriage to Lydia Lopokova.[4] Since Bloomsbury contains one of the most complex relationships in literary history (in which Vanessa Bell's daughter Angelica Garnett is the result of Vanessa's union with Duncan Grant, the one-time lover of Angelica's husband, David Garnett), it is perhaps little wonder that few biographers felt brave enough to face the challenge of explaining and revealing the patterns of friendship within this network. Brave or not, the conventions of biography prior to the mid-1960s were such that revelation, and *telling all*, was not the imperative which it has since become.

But Holroyd did reveal, and he did document, and readers of his lengthy and extensively referenced biography were left in little doubt about the precise details of sexual relations within Lytton Strachey's circle. What, of course, is a more problematic issue is the question of what more we know, in any real sense, by 'knowing' the details of the sexual behaviour of a small (if influential) group of people in English cultural history. But know we do, and as a result of the shift in expectations, the biographer is now expected to tell all, and the reader is expected to want to know. We are no longer left alone with our fantasies, our conjectures and guesses about individual people; the 'colouring in' is done for us. At the same time as biographers have discovered new limits, so too have publishers, and those who control publishing. New boundaries have been set, and new 'permissions' granted to authors of auto/biography. Inevitably, not all those 'permissions' have been mutually agreed: the most notorious case of the shifting of boundaries has been that of the Murdoch press and its revelations about the British Royal Family. Rupert Murdoch, for reasons which can be read as inspired republicanism or frantic desire for profit, was determined to change the boundaries surrounding the behaviour of members of the Royal Family. To a generation brought up within the confines of the complacent reporting of the tranquil home life of 'our own dear Queen', Murdoch's style was radically different. In the early 1970s reporting of the royal family was, at its most dramatic, a picture of the Queen looking cross or Princess Anne falling off her horse. By the mid-1990s members of the royal household had been pictured almost naked on the front page of newspapers and confessed to adultery on television. The fact that more than one member of the Royal Family did these things only served to emphasise Murdoch's point: what was involved in discreet reporting was not the protection of just one morally incompetent individual (in the grand tradition of Edward VII and Edward VIII) but the protection of a whole family of people who were as over-privileged as they were morally dubious.

So what Murdoch demonstrated was the rich possibility of uniting an irreproachable moral campaign, in the revelation of over-privileged hypocrisy, with a vast increase in the profitability of his media empire. Everyone in the media has always known that sensational revelations sell newspapers – the salacious press existed long before the *Sun* or the *Sunday Sport*. But the extent of possible revelation has changed and shifted in the past two hundred years. Attacks on the Royal Family are nothing new (scurrilous cartoons about the sons of George III, were, for example, commonplace), but the degree of permission about reporting has constantly shifted and changed, and changed in response to the engagement of individuals with the press as well as the press with individuals. In Chapter 3, the relationship of the British Royal Family to auto/biography is discussed in greater detail; suffice it to say in this context that it would be premature to assume that the late Princess of Wales was the first member of the Royal Family to engage actively with the mass media.

So the first change that we can see in the recent development of auto/biography is a move towards the inclusion of more information about what is often described as the 'private' life of individuals. The second change that is discernible – and again very much part of recent literary history – is the subject of auto/biography. Although 'diaries of a nobody' (to borrow a title from explicit fiction) have been part of the tradition of auto/biography for some time,[5] in general the subject of auto/biography was a member of a social and/or political elite. When Lytton Strachey published his first best-selling work of biography it was called *Eminent Victorians*, and the title captured precisely the expectations and the assumptions of the genre.[6] Even if we can now read the title ironically and recognise that Strachey was deeply sceptical about the normative system that elevated a General Gordon to 'eminence', we can also recognise that it did not occur to Strachey to write about the men who were with Gordon at Khartoum or to document their experiences or seek their own documentation of experience. Nevertheless, by the time that *Eminent Victorians* was published, the beginnings of the democratic implications of mass literacy were more than evident. Working-class women and men had begun to record their histories, and those members of the middle class who found themselves – through war or personal circumstance – in humble situations had also added their contributions to the historical record. As an example the memoirs of men who fought in the First World War are significant. Few previous wars had seen the reaction in print of the 1914–18 war; from all sides both fictional and non-fictional accounts documented the horrors of the mass slaughter of the trenches.[7] Over and over again, what these accounts emphasised was the commonplace, the shared, nature of this experience. The misery, the ever-present risk of death and mutilation were emphasised as the general, rather than the specific, experience of this war.

The literary impact of the First World War continues to this day. But what is notable in the context of a history of auto/biography is that it marks the clearest indication to that point of the development in English literature of interest in the lives and experiences of ordinary people, involved in but far removed from the decision-making of political events. As historians have now recognised, wars are often a vehicle for social change, and in the history of the development of auto/biography, the First World War was precisely that kind of phenomenon.[8] Even though the best-known accounts of life in the trenches or the hospitals were written by members of gentry or middle-class families (such as Siegfried Sassoon and Vera Brittain) these accounts were nevertheless about commonplace, ordinary experiences.[9] Although from privileged backgrounds, Sassoon and Brittain both had to learn the reality of being commanded by others, and it is this sense of being ruled, of being subject, which is such an evocative part of their accounts. At the same time, what they – and others – gave to auto/biography was the permission to others to write of the mundane and unexceptionable. Hence, in the 1920s and the 1930s there came about a massive interest in the documentary, and the recording of the lives of those who could not record their own experiences. On unemployed men, the poverty-stricken wives and mothers of the Depression, and the veterans of the Civil War in Spain there exists a rich documentary literature.[10] Often the voices of these experiences are confused (and confusing) in that middle-class people take on the responsibility for recording the lives of the less privileged. For example, Orwell's *The Road to Wigan Pier* and *Down and Out in Paris and London* are essentially accounts of a visitor to the lives of the poor.[11]

Nevertheless, for all the problems that Orwell's work contains, we can now recognise it as part of a development within literature of the recognition of the importance of recording the diversity and subjectivity of human experience. Women, as well as men, began to speak of their lives, and the politics of socialism and feminism drew on documentary accounts of the lives of individuals. What Raphael Samuel has described as 'unofficial knowledge' became part of the understanding of our culture and an essential part (on all sides of the political spectrum) of our understanding of the way in which our society works. As Samuel argues, the sources open to historians have recently enlarged considerably:

> The discovery of printed ephemera and its incorporation into library holdings and museum display – a phenomenon of the 1960s – has sensibly enlarged the notion of the historical, turning the spotlight of inquiry on to subjects which would have fallen beneath the dignity of the subject in the past. Who could be interested in a *laundry* list? the eminent Edwardian historian Sir Paul Vinogradov allegedly exclaimed, giving to the term something of the scorn which Lady Bracknell visited on the idea of someone being spawned in a *handbag*.[12]

The boundaries of history, as Samuel goes on the demonstrate, have become wider and less exclusive, to include not just the written record about the lives of the rich and the powerful, but also the artefacts and the literature of the 'ordinary' person.

The reclamation of the past by those outside the circle of the great and good has been one of the more striking features of the cultural history of the twentieth century. That reclamation is, of course, ideally not just a voyage back into the history of a particular group, but equally a reclamation of the present. Whatever we may wish to say about the past, it cannot be relived, whereas the reinterpretation of history, the recognition of marginal, disenfranchised and powerless groups can serve to empower in the present. Thus women, gay people of both sexes, people outside the white, middle and upper class have learned, and valued, their own history as a way to understanding the present. In this context, a new auto/biography has emerged in which the unnamed and the unknown become the central characters of works of recovery. Flora Thompson's *Lark Rise to Candleford* is one instance of a book which caught the public imagination: recollections of the grim and poverty-stricken countryside of late Victorian England were softened by an elegiac prose style, and the success of the author in establishing herself as a member of the salaried middle class.[13] Less muted in its tone was Liz Stanley's reconstruction of the diaries of the nineteenth-century servant woman Hannah Cullwick.[14] There was nothing exceptional about Hannah Cullwick's situation, but there was a great deal that was exceptional about her response to it, in that she wrote (between 1854 and 1873) extensive diaries and recorded not just her daily life, but also the complexity of her relationship with her position and with her employer, Arthur Munby, whom she eventually married. As Liz Stanley writes of her:

> Hannah Cullwick was to a large degree an 'unsexed' woman, one who was loosened although not freed from the fetters of middle class and dependent womanhood, but also one who had determined not to enter working class married womanhood and consequent control over her person by an individual man. She struggled to piece together a 'language' – in her case not only conceptual but literal, in terms of the practical difficulties of communicating at a basic level with Munby as the denizen of a different, although contiguous social milieu – in which to speak and write of this.[15]

We cannot know what Hannah Cullwick would have thought about this (or any other) interpretation of her life.[16] As it is, she emerges in Stanley's account as an assertive and – in Stanley's words – 'as proficient a theoriser of her own and other people's experience as any contemporary feminist theoretician'.[17] This

particular woman and the diaries she left have been reclaimed
by feminism, and incorporated into a theoretical vision which
assumes the endless negotiation between women and men of
social and personal power. Thus Cullwick becomes an instance,
and example, of a particular interpretation of the past (and
indeed the present). Nor is Cullwick the only woman (or person)
who is received into the ready niche of a version of history. In
gay history, and in the history of relations between black and
white in the United States, there are now numerous examples of
individuals who are used to illustrate particular aspects of history
and the historical process. In this exercise, it is both the ordinary
and the extraordinary event which appears: the uneventful life
becomes as worthy of notice as the chronicle of the individual
who has lived through massively dramatic or traumatic events.[18]

It is thus that, in the last decade of the twentieth century, we
can observe the democratisation of auto/biography. The lives of
the great and good are still with us, and these lives still chronicle
the interaction of the great and the good with each other. (Thus,
for example, at least in Britain, there is a high degree of similarity
between the memoirs of many politicians.) But at the same time
as these tomes occupy shelf space, so do the increasingly detailed
and revelatory accounts of the lives of less well known individuals. We are told about their childhoods, their sexual lives and
often – in ghosted autobiographies – given more than rich information about their commercial of professional interactions. In
these diverse auto/biographies there are, inevitably, critical
assessments about the hierarchical 'worth' of works of auto/
biography: there is 'popular' auto/biography (for example of
sportsmen and sportswomen), and there is 'serious', critically
reviewed auto/biography. For the reader, there is now an enormous amount of material about other people's lives and deaths.
Thus we know, courtesy of Andrew Motion, how Philip Larkin
spent his last living hours.[19] Few boundaries remain which have
not been crossed by the zealous biographer or the determined
autobiographer. But in knowing more, in literal and factual
senses, questions need to be asked about the nature of that

knowledge and the relationship of the genre of auto/biography to the world of late twentieth-century capitalism. Furthermore, for all its emancipatory and democratising impulses, we need to ask if the extension and development of auto/biography has limited, rather than extended, human understanding of both the general and the individual self. These possibilities are, perhaps, worth considering as an alternative to an uncritical acceptance of the 'new' auto/biography.

In putting forward a reading of auto/biography which will, I hope, suggest both the problems and the strengths of the genre, the first strand in the argument is the location and definition of the context of auto/biography. In this work, the main focus is auto/biography published in Britain in the last hundred years. As any history of auto/biography states, the genre is considerably older, but as far as this account is concerned, particular qualities of auto/biography emerge in the late nineteenth and early twentieth century which make works of this period definitively different from previous examples of the genre. In brief, these qualities are: the development of self-consciousness, which is a characteristic of early modernism, and the increasingly problematic negotiation of the boundaries between the public and the private. Parallel to these changes in auto/biography are two crucial changes in the context of auto/biography: the emergence of the mass media and individually famous figures within popular culture, and – last but emphatically not least – changes in the definition of gender and racial boundaries. All these characteristics have to be situated, in their turn, within a society which, in Britain after 1900, is urban and industrial but with deep fault lines persisting between classes, races and genders. It was, moreover, a society with an active imperial presence: 'primitive' colonisation was being replaced, by 1900, by a far more systematic organisation of the overseas empire. With this went, as writers about Britain's colonial past have pointed out, an active attempt both to construct and to maintain the 'British' person, a person to set against the non-white, non-British subjects of the empire.[20] In this process of the definition of the British, auto/biography played its part, and from all shades of the political spectrum we can find, by 1935, accounts of being British while living and working in the empire. The idea of 'difference', which was to become a central part of gay and feminist writing in the 1980s and 1990s, was also part of the understanding which informed accounts (such as those by Orwell or Leonard Woolf) of their lives as colonial servants.[21] These men – both part of left/liberal traditions and active in socialist politics – were forced to confront, through their own experiences as colonial servants, the implication of being both different and more powerful in cultures which were not their own.

But the British did not just write auto/biography because of the impact on individuals of the empire. Anglo-Saxon cultures and Protestant cultures in particular, have arguably always had a closer affinity with the auto/biographical form. Protestantism, as critics from Weber onwards have noted, places a heavier burden of responsibility on the individual. In *The Protestant Ethic and the Spirit of Capitalism*, Weber outlined the full psychological impact of Calvinism on the individual :

> The god of Calvinism demanded of his believers not single good works, but a life of good works combined into a unified system. There was no place for the very human Catholic cycle of sin, repentance, atonement, release followed by renewed sin ... The moral conduct of the average man was thus deprived of its planless and unsystematic character and subjected to a consistent method for conduct as a whole.[22]

In the spiritual loneliness of Protestantism (and Calvinism in particular), individuals are removed from the possibility of confession, and explicit forgiveness. There is, in Calvinism, a constant individual gamble on the existence of salvation. None of the mediations of Catholicism (confession, prayers to the saints, the alternative presence to the patriarchal God in the person Virgin Mary) are there for Protestants. In no immediate sense does this order of the religious world account for the emergence of auto/biography, the connection is not as explicit or as direct. But what this model of the symbolic order does create is a need for confession in other forms than those of the expressly religious, as well as a need for personal legitimation and the demonstration of life lived, not as a series of events, but as a project directed towards the possibility of salvation. In his study of the tragedies of Racine and the philosophy of Pascal, *The Hidden God*, Lucien Goldmann suggested the concept of what he described as 'world visions' – the product of a collective consciousness which reaches the highest expression in the mind (and work) of a particular individual.[23] What links the two – world vision and collective consciousness – is seen by Goldmann in terms of coherence, and similarity, at the level of abstraction rather than empirical coincidence. Thus, in *The Hidden God*, Goldmann links the structure and resolution of Racine's tragedies with the actual social and intellectual situation of the social group to which, in seventeenth-century France, Racine belonged. The group to which Racine belonged was known as the *noblesse de robe*; Jansenist in its religious affiliation, it consisted of legal officers who had been granted patents of nobility. But changes in the internal organisation of the French state (as well as religious belief) were increasingly marginalising the *noblesse de robe* and producing, among its members, a sense of separation from the traditional order of society, which they had taken for granted. Central to these changes were increasingly secular expectations about society and community. As Goldmann puts it:

> The rationalism which, when carried to its logical though extreme conclusion, sees men only as isolated individuals for whom other men exist only as objects, also carries out a similar change in man's way of looking at the external world. On the human level, it destroys the idea of community and replaces it by that of an infinitely large collection of reasonable individuals who are all equal and all inter-changeable.[24]

The spiritual bleakness and isolation of post-Reformation and post-Enlightenment Europe is vividly suggested by accounts by those such as Weber and Goldmann. Weber noted the repression of the affective and sensuous elements of European culture, and that insight has been subsequently fully illuminated by feminist historians, who have noted the marginalisation of 'the feminine' (in both literal and symbolic terms) in post-Enlightenment Europe. What has come to hold sway as a major 'world vision' is thus the sense of accountability, of the need for explanation and documentation which are the inevitable results of Calvinism and Protestantism, and which, of course, provide such a fertile breeding-ground for the idea and the development of auto/biography. Deprived of the religious means of literal confession and explanation, the impulse to confess, and to explain oneself (or others) is compelled and channelled into other sources. 'True Confessions', 'I Had to Tell All', these titles from popular culture (even if nowadays inverted with a post-modern sense of irony) carry the weight of the expectations of an earlier European culture which had explicitly allowed the individual to tell all.

But Protestantism removed this possibility from individuals. Thus, at the same time as people (particularly in northern Europe) were becoming more literate and better educated, and cognisant of a more secular, and indeed rational, culture, they were removed from the emotional resource of sharing a sense of responsibility for faults and misdemeanours with those who could help them. It was hardly surprising, therefore, that within the highly individualistic culture of post-Reformation Europe, there was intense interest in individual lives, and lives as models of social possibility. The first literary manifestation of the new interest in the particular individual was the novel, the literary form which – at least in England – is generally associated with the rise of bourgeois individualism.[25] In the novel diverse literary forms came together (the moral tale, the epic, the epistolary), but they had, by the end of the eighteenth century, fused together to produce the great works of early English fiction. The form reached its peak of achievement in the novels of Jane Austen, whose tiny (and deeply self-conscious) canvas nevertheless encompassed the whole range of moral and social issues brought into being by the Enlightenment. Alasdair MacIntyre has elegantly defined Austen as the definitive moralist of modernity, and this judgement speaks volumes about the possibilities of using modernity's definitive form of literature, the novel, to illustrate the general through a study of the particular. In accepting – albeit implicitly – this ideal of fiction, auto/biography accepted the same organising premise as the novel.

In Austen's fiction (and perhaps most fully in *Mansfield Park*) public and private morality are brought together: the boundaries between the household and the world outside are dissolved, and the individual is assumed to be capable of a definitive moral presence. Edward Said has attacked the social vision of *Mansfield Park* (on the grounds of its alleged refusal of a discussion of the exploitative relationship of one of the main characters – Sir Thomas Bertram – with the plantation economies of the West Indies), but that reading, although empirically correct, ignores the substantial assault by Austen on Sir Thomas's 'mercenary' calculations.[26] Austen does not, therefore, launch into an attack on the slave trade, but her attack on the motives behind such relationships is as substantial as any more explicit critique. The problems of the integration of public and private morality are, as Austen is intensely aware, considerable, but she has a unique awareness of the impact on others of behaviour which at first may seem limited and domestic.

Austen did not, of course, write auto/biography, and subsequent biographers have been largely foiled in their zeal by the destruction of many of Austen's letters and papers by her sister Cassandra. But this we have to interpret less as a defence of privacy, in the full contemporary sense, as a defence of something that might be described as the defence of the non-social space in which a person lives. Austen did not defend her privacy, in the sense of concealing actions and thoughts which is now part of late twentieth-century currency, but she made distinctions between actions, and indeed thoughts, which were in some sense the product of thought – indeed rationality – and those which belonged to a different, more spontaneous space. We could, perhaps, regard this space not as 'private' but as 'natural' – a part of the world that is distinct from the culture in which we generally live and share. But as the nineteenth century went on, this space was increasingly colonised by culture, and 'privacy' was constructed as a defence against the inroads of cultural norms into all areas of individual lives. Indeed, by the end of the nineteenth century we can observe that, in many ways and in many contexts, an individual's 'private' life has become synonymous with their sexual practice. Victorian codes about sexuality both repressed and exaggerated sexuality; increasingly, the most powerful were allowed 'private' sexuality, while the least powerful (or less powerful) had their lives policed by a new army of state and institutional guardians of morality.

Thus by the beginning of the twentieth century, we can observe in England, and in North America and parts of northern Europe, a public refusal to discuss, in public, certain aspects of individual lives. Auto/biography throughout the nineteenth century seldom moved outside a rigid record of facts and information. The paucity of the information provided was matched only by the limited number of works published within the genre. But literary modernism brought with it, from the beginning of the twentieth century onwards, a new interest in subjectivity. Numerous feminist scholars have noted the sexual (and indeed cultural) anarchy of the early twentieth century. Elaine Showalter has written of the confusion of gender roles epitomised by reactions to the death of George Eliot ('Queen George' as Showalter describes her). Showalter argues thus:

> The confusion over gender roles at Eliot's funeral reflected her anomalous and crucial position in Victorian letters. George Eliot, whose real name was Marian Evans, had played virtually every role of Victorian gender herself. On the feminine side, as one critic observed, 'she had created herself first as a daughter, then as a sister, and finally as a

mother figure for countless younger men.' Yet the masculine pseudonym, the masculine authority she commanded as a writer, and the range of her intellectual, philosophical, and scientific interests also placed her in the role of father.[27]

Reactions to Eliot's death were (appropriately) diverse. Precisely because Eliot had been so intensely engaged in the general intellectual debates of her time – and debates largely structured and organised by men – she had established a norm of participation in masculinised aspects of the culture with which it was difficult for some women to sympathise. Indeed, Eliot's own well-known attacks on 'silly novels by lady novelists' had set her own standards about what was significant in literature.[28] Many women writing in the period immediately after Eliot's death had happily mocked Eliot's standards: the greater self-confidence in the specifically 'female' voice which emerges in this period carried with it a delegitimatisation of the values about the novel (and indeed the culture generally) that Eliot espoused.

Hence, from women writers – and indeed from homosexual men who wished to escape the normative expectations of Victorian male heterosexuality – came a new voice: a voice that asserted subjectivity and diversity, and eschewed the apparently objective aspirations of Eliot and her followers. The clearest examples of this shift were to be found in Proust, Joyce and Woolf, writers who had little truck with the great Victorian attempts at the comprehensive explanation of social life in literature. Their concern was the evocation of individual experience, not the weighty discussion of the relationship between the individual and society which characterises Eliot. The tensions created by this shift, often defined in terms of a shift away from social realism in fiction, continue to this day. But it is the impact of these shifts on auto/biography that is of concern here, and of that impact it can be said that the results were – by the 1920s – becoming glaringly apparent. The most explicit movement away from the conventional Victorian auto/biography was made by Lytton Strachey in 1918, with the publication of *Eminent*

Victorians. (It is ironic that, just as Strachey himself made radical changes in auto/biography, so too did biographical writing about Strachey.) The work was appropriately published in the year in which the end of the First World War brought with it the end of Victorian England, and the Europe of the old dynastic empires. Bourgeois society continued, but the particular form of bourgeois society that was created by Victorian morality and the impact of imperialism was lost forever. Strachey's biographer, Michael Holroyd, wrote of Strachey's subjects:

> His polemic against Cardinal Manning is an attack on the evangelicalism that was to be a defining characteristic of nineteenth-century culture, an exposure of its hypocrisy and the emptiness of self-regarding ambitions. In toppling Florence Nightingale from the pedestal where she posed as the legendary lady with the lamp, saintly and self-sacrificing, and replacing her with a twentieth-century neurotic, Strachey struck directly at the popular mythology of Victorian England, in particular its conscious saving humanitarianism. His enmity towards the third eminent Victorian, Dr Arnold, probably arose from his own unhappy schooldays. He depicts Arnold as the most influential teacher of the Victorians. His target was not only the public school system, the cult of which stultified middle-class intelligence and set hard the ethos of Victorianism into the twentieth century, but the whole movement of nineteenth-century liberalism based not on the principles of progress but on a variation of old and debased routines. Finally, he shows us General Gordon indulging his secret passion for fame and becoming a willing instrument not of God but of the extreme imperialist faction of the British Government.[29]

In retrospect, we can see that what Strachey achieved in *Eminent Victorians* was the modernisation of auto/biography. Strachey and the circle within which he moved were well aware of the work of Freud, and of the possibilities of psychoanalysis. In this knowledge, Strachey and his contemporaries had a supremely effective weapon with which to attempt to reveal the reality behind public façades. 'Creative destruction', which David Harvey has described as typical of cultural modernism,[30] is an apt summary for Strachey's *magnum opus*, in that Strachey took away, and deconstructed, the myths surrounding his subjects and replaced them with alternative models of interpretation. For example, in his conclusion to the section on Florence Nightingale, Strachey wrote: 'The terrible commander who had driven Sidney Herbert to his death, to whom Mr Jowett had applied the words of Homer – raging insatiably – now accepted small compliments with gratitude, and indulged in sentimental friendships with young girls.'[31] As Holroyd notes, Strachey's eye for hypocrisy and self-serving was never less than acute, and throughout *Eminent Victorians* there was a powerful sub-text of scepticism about the public virtues of Victorian England.

Eminent Victorians was an immediate success with the reading public, and marks a watershed in the genre of auto/biography. But this assessment is made retrospectively, and the transformation of the possibilities of auto/biography was hardly immediately apparent. Indeed, there is a considerable case to argue that the transformation is still incomplete, and that just as literary modernism remains a disputed form of fiction, so 'modern' auto/biography remains only one form of possibility among others. While Strachey offered a model of writing which suggested an interpretation of an individual, we can also see traditions at work in twentieth-century auto/biography – both organised around different relationships, and different positions, *vis-à-vis* modernism. Thus there is (and always has been) the rigidly 'objective' auto/biography which maintains a sealed belief in the 'facts' of the case and refuses anything approaching subjectivity. The memoirs of most politicians and biographies of the great and the good tend to fall into this category: the idea that politicians might be motivated by the same inadequacies that made General Gordon frantic for fame is not entirely integrated into the understanding of those who have devoted their lives to the maintenance of conservatism with either a large or small first letter. Characteristic of this form of the genre is a refusal of the discussion of childhood (which might, of course, have something to say about the nature of the adult person) and the marginalisation of anything relating to emotional life. In this, biographers refuse their own understanding as much as the reader's understanding of the subject. For example, in his biography of Harold Macmillan, Alasdair Horne referred to the long-standing relationship between Lady Dorothy Macmillan (Macmillan's aristocratic wife) and Lord Boothby.[32] The relationship was a well-known aspect of the Macmillan's life, and one of those open secrets of metropolitan politics. Yet – as Horne points out – at no time did Macmillan himself refer to it or consider the implications. More surprising still, since we may conjecture that Macmillan, for his own reasons (whether of hurt or lack of interest), did not wish to discuss the matter, was Horne's failure to connect this silence with Macmillan's behaviour in the Profumo scandal of 1963. Faced with the possibility of a sexual scandal in which national security interests were involved, and the consequent need to investigate personal and sexual relationships, Macmillan simply refused to act.

This double denial – first by Macmillan, and second by Horne – is characteristic of a great deal of the auto/biographical tradition that has refused the implications and possibilities of modernism. In this and other examples, what we can see at work particularly clearly is that rigid invocation of the distinction between the public and the private which has long been a characteristic of aspects of, and interests within, bourgeois society. In the early nineteenth century there was, as already suggested in the case of the novels of Jane Austen, a determination to integrate the public and the private. The loss of privilege implicit in this view was not lost on many people; inevitably, it was a deeply contested issue throughout the nineteenth century and rapidly acquired a gendered focus as women asserted their opposition to the double standard of sexual morality. This opposition, voiced in the campaign over the Contagious Diseases Acts of the 1860s and throughout campaigns for the education and enfranchisement of women, asserted that private behaviour was as important in the assessment of a person's (usually a man's) character as their behaviour in public.[33] The idea was endorsed by the values of Queen Victoria and the Prince Consort; at the same time it was widely ignored and flouted by many of their subjects, not least their oldest son. What is emphasised in traditional biographies of Edward VII (most strikingly Sir Philip Magnus) is the idea that, while Edward VII flouted all expectations of fidelity within marriage, he did so with perfect decorum and with immaculate concern for his wife. Thus Magnus praises Edward VII for his inspired management of those boundaries between the public and the private which allowed Edward to enjoy serial adultery.[34]

The example of Edward VII, while suggesting much that is interesting about the history of the British Royal Family, is also important in that it demonstrates that negotiation of public and private which is so crucial to biography. At the same time it also illuminates the reasons why auto/biography is often seen as a genre which privileges given social hierachies; we know the history of Edward VII better than we know the history of Queen Alexandra or the royal mistresses. It is not that biographies of these women do not exist, it is more that the control of the central narrative is with the author of the auto/biography of Edward VII and thus, implicitly, with Edward VII himself. This does, of course, reflect with some accuracy the power relations between Edward VII and his female significant others, yet in that refection there is often an unspoken endorsement of the values of the more powerful. Here, then, is auto/biography as a form of the protection of the status quo – the assumption that what can be taken for granted is hierarchical power and its impact on individuals. Inevitably, given this form of auto/biography, there has been a very considerable energy behind those works of auto/biography that are designed to reveal the histories of those who are apparently less powerful or even marginal. In this light too, it is less surprising that individuals who cannot control the conventional organisation of auto/biography will resort to 'tell all' auto/ biography. Marginalised by the accounts of the powerful, they have little recourse (other than silence) except through disclosure.

Throughout the nineteenth and twentieth centuries the tensions between public and private continued. In this context, what is essentially at stake is the control of the narrative of individual experience and individual subjectivity, a control which is generally (although not always) located in those who are most powerful. At the same time, the powerful are imprisoned within a perception of the construction of the self, which often has both a negative and a distorting impact on the accounts given. That construction of the self which informs auto/biography is complex, but can be described in terms of a number of assumptions, all shared throughout the contemporary West. One such assumption is the belief that we are an integrated 'individual' self, with a coherent persona. Despite considerable psychoanalytic (and indeed empirical) evidence to the contrary, the social expectation – increasingly enforced by the culture and the demands of the labour market – is that we are a 'knowable' person, a person with a coherent emotional *curriculum vitae* For many individuals, the demands of being this kind of stable, never-changing self are impossible. Nevertheless, what auto/biography often tends to endorse is the view that the 'real' person can be identified and presented to the reading public. What Lytton Strachey was content to do in biography was to interpret a life: indeed *Eminent Victorians*, and his later *Elizabeth and Essex* and *Queen Victoria*, are essentially modern essays in 'reading' a life. There is all the difference in the world between this confident interpretation and other works of the twentieth century (for example Philip Ziegler on Mountbatten)[35] which assume that, in the collection and presentation of all available material about a subject, coherence will emerge. What we can see at work here is a sense of the subject (that is, the self of both subject studied and author of the study) which has a strongly internalised sense of the possibility of defining and knowing the individual.

What goes with this view is an equally powerful tacit under-standing of human lives as lived according to a narrative model, in which our hero or heroine sets out on a journey, is educated through the events of his or her life, and reaches a point of reconciliation with circumstance. I would therefore propose here that what auto/biography often cannot do is to sever its links with narrative fiction. When Henry Fielding wrote *Tom Jones*, or Dickens *Oliver Twist* and *Nicholas Nickleby*, they created accounts of human life which have become paradigms of general assump-tions about the organisation of experience. As such, it is often impossibly difficult for authors of auto/biography to distinguish between facts about individuals and powerful fictional stereo-types. Moreover, having failed to make this basic distinction, it is also the case that authors of auto/biography cannot appreciate the impact of fiction on fact; that is, the sense in which indi-viduals create themselves in relationship to a fantasy. For instance, in the discussion of de Beauvoir in Chapter 2, there is an example of a woman who created herself in relation to certain characters in fiction. It is this kind of blurring of the lines between fact and fiction that can make auto/biography so unreliable, at the same time as it can reduce literally minded critics to apoplexy at the thought that 'facts' are being confused with 'fiction'.

The prison created by the need for the coherent self has one further aspect which should be noted here. It is that, just as the authors of biographies impose (or attempt to impose) order on the lives of the subjects, so authors of autobiographies often become the prisoners, even in the presentation of their lives, of over-determined, and over-determining forces among which a sense of rigid chronology is only one example. When George Eliot asked the question in *Daniel Deronda* about where to start a narrative, she asked a question which might even be asked in auto/biography. Indeed, the most powerful works of auto/biography in the twentieth century have been written outside conventional chronological organisation. Jean Paul Sartre's *Words* was an explicit refusal by the author of the ordinary expectations of autobiography.[36] Unlike his life-long friend, Simone de Beau-voir, Sartre took the dominating motif of his life and made that the basis of his account of his life. In doing so, he produced a work which arguably gave a more accurate account of his life than the thousands of words produced by de Beauvoir. The extent to which her autobiography illustrates the limits and eva-sions of the form as conventionally interpreted will be the subject of the next chapter.

Chapter 2

Lies, all lies
Auto/biography as fiction

If the self in modernity is more fractured than in previous historical periods, the impulse by many writers has been to try to heal that sense of fragmentation by embracing documentation and emphatically chronological narrative. Of all the people, both women and men, writing in the West in the twentieth century, Simone de Beauvoir is a paradigmatic illustration of a person anxious to maintain, through the written word, a sense of herself as a coherent person. De Beauvoir's global fame is largely a product of her association with feminism, particularly the publication in 1949 of *The Second Sex*. As with other cases of considerable fame, the association is not entirely accurate: there is no doubt that de Beauvoir was the author of *The Second Sex*, but her relationship to feminism was rather more tangential, and more a product of feminism's discovery of de Beauvoir than an original commitment on de Beauvoir's part.[1]

From her account of her childhood and adolescence, we are told de Beauvoir was always determined to be a writer. She regarded words, as is clear from the account she gives of her early life, as crucially important and as the means through which she would negotiate and establish her adult, autonomous self. That she did this is now part of history, and when de Beauvoir died in 1986 she left behind a considerable volume of written work: fiction, autobiography and essays in philosophy. All this writing is marked by a commitment and adherence to the conventional

forms of narrative: de Beauvoir begins her autobiography literally at the beginning, with her birth and brief portraits of her
parents. Her novels have the same chronological organisation,
and even when they are relatively brief and written as first-
person narratives (as in the case of her two late novels, *Les Belles
Images* and *The Woman Destroyed*), they are nevertheless conventionally organised and the character's sense of self presented
as part of a recognisable and fixed form.[2] Her novels all present
cases of intense human (particularly female) suffering, but that
suffering is the more intense precisely because it is presented as a
result of a challenge to fixed definitions of self. For example, the
central female character in *The Woman Destroyed* suffers agonies of
misery because of her husband's affair with a younger woman.
Upsetting and disturbing as the affair is, it is apparent that what is
threatening about this is the disturbance it presents to an ordered
and predictable set of events. Equally, de Beauvoir returns in *The
Woman Destroyed* to the theme which has been present in her
previous novels; the ability of men to arouse in women sexual
jealousy and threaten a sense of self organised around heterosexual relationships.

This intense identification by women with male others – and
indeed the achievement of happiness through this form of relationship – is a theme which dominates de Beauvoir's fiction, quite
as much as it clearly dominated her own life. To read de Beauvoir's novels today is to step back into a world in which authors
took for granted bourgeois, heterosexual expectations about sexual relationships. Indeed, despite her radical credentials and her
espousal of left-wing causes, much of de Beauvoir's fiction is
organised within an entirely conventional construct: the exploration of the moral problems of heterosexual relationships, an
exploration which would not have been out of place in the novels
of Eliot or Tolstoy. Dominating the fiction is a sense of the possibility of an absolute morality, a morality for 'all seasons' that was
to be deposed by post-modernist espousals of moral pluralism.
Despite her links to existentialism, which at least theoretically
allows the individual space for moral negotiation, de Beauvoir

pursued to the end of life a fixedly modern belief in the possibility of the definitive explanation. *The Second Sex* had outlined a
thesis about women which constructed gender relations in terms
of opposition (male/female and men/women); *Old Age* was to do
the same for the idea of becoming old (the old versus the young).
Entirely absent from these theoretical constructs was any sense of
the ambiguities possible within definitions of male and female,
young and old.[3]

These brief remarks about de Beauvoir are made in order to
give some sense of the work of a woman who, despite the evident
qualifications in the passages above, nevertheless has a com-
manding place in twentieth-century intellectual history. However,
it is the contention of this chapter that de Beauvoir occupies this
place less because of the strength of her accounts and explanations of the social and intellectual worlds than through her central symbolic presence, which she largely constructed for herself,
as an autonomous woman. To continue this argument, what de
Beauvoir represents within our particular culture is a female version of Prometheus Unbound. As symbols of the possibilities of
male intellectual strength and liberation in European bourgeois
culture there are numerous male candidates; until de Beauvoir,
there have been very few, if any, women who could claim the
same iconographic status. The great woman writers of the nineteenth century often went out of their way to define themselves
as secure (and secured) inhabitants of a domestic space. Even
George Eliot (and perhaps particularly George Eliot, precisely
because of the moral and social ambiguities of her position *vis-à-
vis* George Lewes) explicitly rejected modes of female emancipation which seemed to suggest personal and sexual autonomy. To
be part of the culture, to occupy a defining space within that
culture, it seemed to be necessary for women to emphasise, if not
actually exaggerate, their endorsement of the values of domesticity and the household.[4] What women did with this domestic
space was, of course, to make it into the place from which they
launched passionate attacks on the conventional organisation of
womanhood. When Charles Dickens wrote of Elizabeth Gaskell

that, if he was Mr Gaskell, 'how he would beat her', he caught some of the sense of male impotence when confronted by the powerful pens of women who turned the domestic hearth into a radical, critical space.[5]

But de Beauvoir was to move intellectual, and intellectually engaged, women into another mode. Informed by the literature of nineteenth-century Britain and the United States (Jo of *Little Women* and Maggie Tulliver in *The Mill on the Floss* are mentioned by de Beauvoir as important, influential characters), de Beauvoir recognised the possibilities of literature for her own form of female emancipation. The authors of *Little Women* and *The Mill on the Floss* are now instantly recognisable as powerful female voices: in choosing to identify with them, de Beauvoir placed herself directly in line with that assertive female tradition. Nevertheless, what she was also to do was to carry into her work, albeit in an entirely unacknowledged and unrevealed form, all the inconsistencies and ambiguities of Alcott and Eliot. Like them, she spoke in ways that took much from conventional, 'masculine' fiction, and like them she never managed to break away from the seductive possibilities of masculinity. In this, therefore, her work represents one of the most complex accounts of femininity in the twentieth century although it is a paradox of the work that it is only a conventional understanding of feminism which can read de Beauvoir as a feminist. Her presence as a radical figure has been agreed by Toril Moi, but against this can be set a considerable evidence that suggests the essentially conservative and conventional nature of de Beauvoir's work.[6] Not the least aspect of this essential conservatism is de Beauvoir's highly literal understanding of the world and social relationships, and her deeply ambiguous attitude to the subjectivity of others. In short – and the summary of the discussion to follow – what de Beauvoir represents is the autonomous female heroine of bourgeois society, and one who explicitly used auto/biography as a means of constructing that self. It was a presence constructed in part by de Beauvoir herself (in the face of the full knowledge of the reality of the experience of others) but also in part drawn from the

expectations of a society which sees intellectual life in highly
personal terms, terms which are structured by and related to a
system of hierarchical achievement.

Obviously, these are grave comments (if not accusations) to
make about a woman regarded in some quarters as the greatest
heroine of twentieth-century feminism. But, as Brecht tellingly
remarked, we should always be wary of the land which has a
need for heroes. The 'land' of feminism is extensive, but the
Western version of feminism, particularly the feminism of the
white United States, has long endorsed female achievement in
male spheres. In this model, De Beauvoir is an excellent example
of achievement: a successful novelist, an acclaimed philosopher,
and the author of a best-selling (and highly influential) account
of the condition of women. Although her radical politics have
attracted attention (not least in her native France at the time of
the Algerian war of independence), such is the organisation of de
Beauvoir's work that its potentially disruptive radicalism is effectively compartmentalised from de Beauvoir, the author of *The
Second Sex* and volumes of autobiography. Anyone reading the
conclusion to *The Second Sex* would have little difficulty in fitting
de Beauvoir into the most conventional model of Western
achievement. Although the book provides a telling account of
Western misogyny (and is organised in a way which was to
inspire, among others, Kate Millett and Shulamith Firestone),
the conclusion suggests the thesis of integration into this society,
rather than any radical change of it.[7] It is the argument replicated a thousand times in campaigns to change the nature of
institutions by including more women in them. It is, as such,
an argument which depends upon a certain essentialism and a
limited understanding of the power of institutions to mould
and influence human behaviour.[8]

But an understanding of the complexities of social life and
social relations is not a defining characteristic of de Beauvoir's
work. The elder daughter of a French bourgeois family, she was
brought up within a rigid structure of manners and behaviour, a
structure which was constantly undermined by the behaviour of

her father. The first volume of de Beauvoir's autobiography, *Memoirs of a Dutiful Daughter*, describes the happy, sensual days of her childhood, a bliss shattered by the decline in the family's material circumstances and the shift from a prosperous bourgeois existence to a marginal, poverty-stricken existence.[9] The once carefree mother becomes the household drudge, the affectionate father an absent figure, more often to be found in cafés than in his home. This duality of existence – the maintenance of bourgeois form and the equally obvious sub-text of dissolute infidelity – became the dominating organisation of de Beauvoir's adolescence. Her mother took refuge in pious Catholicism, her father in equally fervent secularism. From this, de Beauvoir emerged with a passionate commitment to her apparent means of escape: the competence in ideas and language that would enable her to pass examinations and forge for herself an independent existence.

At the end of the twentieth century it is easy to write these words lightly, without any indication of their meaning in the 1920s. Yet what de Beauvoir did, in taking philosophy examinations and training as a teacher, was not just rare, it was exceptional. Very few women in France (or anywhere else in the West) undertook the work and the commitment necessary to acquire professional qualifications. But de Beauvoir did this because, as we know, the young Simone had to earn her own living, and we know that she wished to be able to live away from home, and away from the rows and the miseries which had come to dominate it. But at the same time we have to ask, why philosophy, and why teaching? What were the motivations and the pressures that directed this person in this particular direction?

It is on this point that we meet the first major absence in de Beauvoir's autobiography, and in doing so have the first example of the pattern of evasions, absences and at times misrepresentations that characterises her autobiography. From *Memoirs of a Dutiful Daughter*, we know that de Beauvoir was attracted to explanations of the world which seemed to offer an alternative to her mother's Catholicism. But the question of belief in God, which was a part of the world view of Enlightenment philosophers, does not enter into de Beauvoir's conception of the world. Indeed, it is possible to 'read' de Beauvoir's first volume of autobiography as a lengthy account of separation from her mother. Embracing philosophy, and the particular understanding of philosophy which de Beauvoir chose, was thus a lengthy engagement with the secularism of her father. Hence, we do not find de Beauvoir troubled by Kant's belief in God, or the work of numerous Enlightenment and post-Enlightenment philosophers on the meaning of God, whether as a literal presence or as a symbolic meaning. What we do find her troubled by is the association of organised religion (and in this de Beauvoir always means French Roman Catholicism) with women. Thus she writes, in *Memoirs*:

> My father was not a believer; the greatest writers and the finest thinkers shared his scepticism; on the whole, it was generally the women who went to church; I began to find it paradoxical and upsetting that the truth should be *their* privilege, when men, beyond all possible doubt, were their superiors.[10]

Several pages follow this comment (which richly deserves close attention for its view of women and men), in which de Beauvoir describes more fully the months in which she gradually lost her faith in God. But then, just as it would seem that she might plunge into an abyss of emptiness, she is saved. What saves her is words: in the first instance the words are those of other people (in this case Louisa M. Alcott and George Eliot), although very soon words as process, as writing, begin to emerge. As she says: 'As soon as I had given up all hopes of heaven, my worldly ambitions increased; I had to get on in life.' And in the following paragraph she develops these remarks by pointing out that she does not wish merely to write but to be a famous author, to climb to 'rarefied spheres' through her own achievements.[11]

This is precisely what de Beauvoir achieved. *Memoirs of a Dutiful Daughter* left de Beauvoir at the threshold of adult life, a graduate of the Sorbonne and a fully accepted and accredited teacher of philosophy. The following two volumes of auto-biography, *The Prime of Life* and *Force of Circumstance* chronicle de Beauvoir's adult life, her engagement with the wider world of intellectual and political events and, above all, the nature of her relationship with Jean-Paul Sartre.[12] Yet in the final volume of her autobiography, *All Said and Done* (published in 1972 and dedi-cated to Sylvie le Bon, the woman with whom de Beauvoir shared the last years of her life), de Beauvoir returns to the issue of God.[13] The heroines of her adolescence return in the final passages of the book, and there is the same explicit and deter-mined rejection of the idea of God that characterised the ado-lescent de Beauvoir. There is no sense of the impossibility of answering the question of the existence of God: what de Beau-voir affirms is her rigid determination not to allow this idea. Instead, it is difficult not to see de Beauvoir creating herself as the God of her own existence. She writes, 'I wanted to make myself exist for others by conveying, as directly as I could, the taste of my own life: I have more or less succeeded.'[14]

There are ancient ideas about graven images which might seem appropriate here, not necessarily from a viewpoint which categorically asserts the existence of God, but from a position which allows the impossibility of the definitive answer to the question. But the difficulty of answering questions about a range of issues, including the existence of God, was not, on the whole, a position that had much appeal for de Beauvoir. Hence, in her autobiography we can hear the constant voice of a woman who wishes to impose her understanding on events, and show the difference between her views and those of others. The motivation could be described as a mania for separation and individuation; implicit and unacknowledged as her mother is, de Beauvoir often uses the 'failure' of others to separate themselves from their parents' (and in particular their mother's) views as the reason for their imperfect understanding. Thus in explaining the difference between her (de Beauvoir's) loss of faith in God and the constant belief of her friend Zaza (Elizabeth Mabille) de Beauvoir writes:

> Zaza had a critical mind and many aspects of her religion puzzled her; yet because of her painful, unconditional love for her mother she did not renounce it – she did not wish to move farther away from her in her own mind.[15]

No such inhibitions prevented de Beauvoir taking up, in her adolescence, a position of determined atheism, a position to which she was faithful throughout her life.

But what she put in the place of a Catholic God was a belief system organised around a literal, human person, in the form of Jean-Paul Sartre. *The Prime of Life*, volume two of the autobiography, begins with the sexual consummation of de Beauvoir's relationship with Sartre, and the account by de Beauvoir of the negotiation between them about the nature of the relationship. In *The Prime of Life* de Beauvoir's account suggests a blissfully happy de Beauvoir receiving Sartre's definition of the situation:

> Sartre was not inclined to be monogamous by nature: he took pleasure in the company of women, finding them less comic than men. He had no intention, at twenty three, of renouncing their tempting variety. He explained the matter to me in his favourite terminology. 'What we have', he said, 'is an *essential* love; but it is a good idea for us also to experience *contingent* love affairs.'[16]

Yet other accounts, including that of de Beauvoir's loyal biographer Deirdre Bair, suggest that the relationship between Sartre and de Beauvoir was full of unresolved tensions, not the least of which was Sartre's enormous enthusiasm for the company of other women and his equally considerable enthusiasm to share those experiences with de Beauvoir.[17]

What emerges from this situation is a less than equal access to sexual revelation. Deirdre Bair, and de Beauvoir herself, relay the accounts which Sartre gave to de Beauvoir of his sexual escapades. In all these cases, de Beauvoir took the position of the good listener; in reality this seems to have been the case, and it is an impression which is certainly conveyed in the autobiography. Although de Beauvoir allows herself to express momentary flashes of jealousy in print, on the whole she maintains the position of concerned onlooker to Sartre's *amours*. But what this does is to create in the reader's mind a picture of de Beauvoir as passive, as the spectator to Sartre's womanising and her obsessive concern with the recall of his sexual conquests. In this (a situation in which de Beauvoir colludes with Sartre's infantile narcissism), de Beauvoir herself is deprived of both emotional and sexual being. The deception is therefore two-fold: in her autobiography, neither does de Beauvoir reveal to us *how* she experienced Sartre's endless infidelity, nor does she fully acknowledge her own sexual feelings or her sexual relations with others. She does, as all readers of the autobiography know, make much of the sexual feelings she experienced at the beginning of the relationship with Sartre, but readers are given no hint, either then or in subsequent pages, that de Beauvoir pursued diverse sexual relationships outside the relationship with Sartre, in terms of both the number and the gender of the individuals involved.

In this creation of a passive autobiographical self, de Beauvoir effectively limits her own agency and leaves an absence in the history of her life which is only now being put together by the reminiscences and revelations of former lovers. The rage, jealousy, fear and envy which could have been a part of her experiences at this time do, however, appear in print in another form, her novels. In *She Came to Stay*, the first of de Beauvoir's novels to be published (although not the first she wrote), she presented an account of a woman driven to murder by the disruption of a fictional relationship very obviously that of de Beauvoir and Sartre.[18] The woman in real life was named Olga Kosakievicz, a pupil of de Beauvoir's during her school teaching days in Rouen and very rapidly the recipient of all the fantasies and ideas which Sartre and de Beauvoir had about themselves. Olga became Sartre's lover, and gradually acquired a position of such importance in his life that de Beauvoir felt herself marginalised. The fictional resolution was *She Came to Stay*, the resolution in reality was de Beauvoir's serious illness and her departure, both physically and emotionally from the trio.

After the many, lasting traumas of the relationship with Olga, de Beauvoir's account of her life with Sartre enters a long period of calm and almost emotional inactivity. In 1939 Sartre was conscripted into the French army and imprisoned. Although eventually freed he was destined to live something of a muted existence in occupied France. The couple did not engage actively in Resistance work of the conventional kind (de Beauvoir and Sartre were not inclined to take up arms), but their work and their interests were sufficiently subversive for them to be able to act less than fully. Censorship was considerable, if patchily and often ineffectively applied. Nevertheless, Sartre's *Being and Nothingness* was published in 1943; its very obscurity no doubt keeping it from the attention of the German censors. For Sartre and de Beauvoir the war years were a time of literary work; as *The Prime of Life* suggests, there was considerable effort involved simply in maintaining daily life, and this, accompanied by the couple's fervent desire to write, engaged the major part of their energies. This, at any rate, is the picture created by *The Prime of Life* – that the war years were years of an almost monastic seclusion, broken only by brief excursions into the French countryside.

The end of the war and the liberation of Paris marked for de Beauvoir and Sartre the beginning of a new period in their lives. By 1945, they had both completed their apprenticeship to literature and become published and well-known authors in France. What the end of the war offered to them was very similar to what it offered to millions of other Europeans: the beginning of a long period of peace, but also a peace dominated by a new form of political relations – the Cold War tensions between East and West and a new form of global culture derived from the United States. Prior to 1939 both Sartre and de Beauvior had known its music, cinema and literature. But until 1945 there was little chance of going there. Now, at the end of the war, first Sartre and subsequently de Beauvoir found themselves much in demand for lecture tours to explain to the citizens of the United States the culture and cultural identity of the newly liberated Europe. With their visits to the United States, both Sartre and de Beauvoir began new and highly significant relationships. In the case of de Beauvoir, the relationship was with the American writer Nelson Algren, in Sartre's case the person involved was known in de Beauvoir's memoirs as 'M'.[19]

These new relationships opened up, in many ways, new worlds for both Sartre and de Beauvoir. Inasmuch as the relationships were part of the new world of the United States, they also demanded of Sartre and de Beauvoir new commitments and new understanding. Here, suddenly, were 'others', those shadowy but essential figures of existentialism who made clear their own demands and their own interpretation of the situation. In the 1930s and the war years, Sartre and de Beauvoir had largely been involved with people known to each other – Olga was the most obvious example of shared involvement, but others shared the attention (sexual and emotional) of both. None of these relationships (with the exception of that with Olga) appear in de Beauvoir's autobiography. Yet after her death, a stream of revelation began, in which ex-lovers put forward their side of the story. For example, in 1996 the woman who appears as Bianca Bienenfeld published her account of her seduction as a sixteen-year-old schoolgirl by de Beauvoir, and one year later by Sartre.[20] De Beauvoir's account of the relationship in *The Prime of Life* notes Bianca's appearance, and her problems of living in Paris as a Jew during the German occupation, but no other significance is recorded.[21]

Thus *The Prime of Life*, and to a large extent *Force of Circumstance*, give accounts of de Beauvoir's life which are, to say the least, selective and highly censored. What is clear from this is that, although de Beauvoir made much of her emancipation from her Catholic, bourgeois background, she was still aware that much of her behaviour would have met, and would probably still meet, censure across a wide range of moral viewpoints. At one end of the moral continuum, bourgeois Catholicism would condemn her completely; other, more liberal attitudes would still regard as problematic the exploitation by two adults of vulnerable adolescents. What emerges therefore, is an autobiography in which de Beauvoir's will to freedom and her expressed, and real, desire for freedom and autonomy, takes the form of the oppression of others. Most particularly, she exhibits a considerable refusal of the subjectivity of others. It is not that de Beauvoir does not express concern about the plight of Bianca and other French Jews, but what is absent is an understanding of the ways in which individual experience of the world is determined by circumstances beyond the control of individuals. The period 1945–50, as presented in her work, thus provides us with a crucial insight into de Beauvoir's understanding of autobiography: she embraces the United States and the post-war world (in both a literal and a symbolic sense), yet at the same time refuses a recognition of modernity – and its implicit moral singularity – imposed by the revelations about the Holocaust. It is a vision that has the essential characteristics of a blinkered perspective: an interpretation locked into a narrow experience of a small group of incestuous individuals in Paris and assuming an uninterrupted continuity between a particular self (or two particular selves in this case) and the assumptions of bourgeois individualism. It is not the case, of course, that de Beauvoir was unaware of the horrors of the 'final solution'. As *Force of Circumstance* makes plain, de Beauvoir was well aware of the existence of Belsen and Auschwitz.[22] Thus what is not at stake here is de Beauvoir's empirical recognition of the Holocaust; rather, it was the theoretical implication of this event which was more problematic. Crucially, what was absent from de Beauvoir's understanding was the realisation that reason, that very God on which she had staked her existence, could create a form of bureaucratic rationality which made possible systematic anti-Semitism.

These are, perhaps, severe accusations to bring against a woman regarded in some quarters as the 'mother' of twentieth-century feminism and the author of an outstanding autobiography. Yet in that ascription lie two issues: the first being our expectations of 'truth' and revelation about autobiographical writing, the second being the receptivity of sections of feminism to de Beauvoir's interpretation of the world. In the first case, the issue of 'truth' in autobiography, it can be said that in looking for this characteristic in autobiography it is all too easy for readers and critics to tie themselves to a highly literal (and imprisoning) construction of veracity. In many ways, and in many instances, we cannot fault de Beauvoir's autobiography as 'untrue' in the sense that she claimed non-existent experiences or friendships. There is no doubt that what she tells us is in a literal sense 'true'. Yet at the same time, this understanding of truth questions the very meaning of the word, in that de Beauvoir leaves out or obscures so much that is of significance. She does not spare the reader the details of her anguish about the problems of her relationship with Nelson Algren, nor her jealousy about Sartre's involvement with Dolores Ehrenreich. But at the same time many others, and their feelings, are not there. This refusal of others and their perception of events may well be an allowable feature of autobiography, but what it provoked, at least in Nelson Algren, was a furious rage at what he perceived as a betrayal of privacy and trust.[23]

The intensity, and the sexual passion, of the affair between Algren and de Beauvoir are evident both from her auto-biography and from her novel *The Mandarins*, large sections of which are thinly disguised accounts of her time in the United States with Algren.[24] As far as Algren was concerned, the rela-tionship was one to which he was fully committed, and fully committed in the conventional heterosexual sense of proposing marriage and domestic life. These expectations were hardly based on a wilful misunderstanding of de Beauvoir's feelings: she spoke of Algren as her 'husband', and the passages in *The Man-darins* in which she describes her life with Algren are written in a form which would not be out of place in a Mills and Boon romance. Thus, for example, she wrote :

There was no need to be upset: he was caressing my hair,

speaking gentle simple words, slipping an old copper ring on my finger. I looked at the ring, listened to those almost forgotten words being spoken in a strange foreign language; under my cheek, I heard the familiar beating of a strange heart. Nothing was asked of me; I had only to be exactly what I was and a man's desire transformed me into a miracle of perfection. It was so restful that if the sun had stopped in the middle of the sky, eternity would have slipped by without my noticing it.[25]

But it was not that de Beauvoir left for fiction what she could not say in fact. She admits, very fully, the degree of her love for Algren and the cost of the relationship to her. Of all the relationships with men which she acknowledged (and these are given in the autobiography as only three – Sartre, Algren and Claude Lanzmann), it is the relationship with Algren which is most forcefully discussed. Sartre is, from the beginning of *The Prime of Life*, omnipresent, but he is assumed as part of de Beauvoir's life and hence often has little emotional presence. It is only when a relationship between Sartre and another woman becomes particularly threatening that Sartre takes on an immediate human reality. Otherwise, he acts as the definitive intellectual arbiter of France and, as he becomes more famous, the world.

For all their length, and lengthy disclosure, the four volumes of de Beauvoir's autobiography are readable as exercises in concealment rather than revelation. The crucial evasions are de Beauvoir's sexual relations with women and men, other than the publicly acceptable figures whom she describes, and (a characteristic of all the volumes of the autobiography) a constant restraint and process of selection in the account she gives of herself and her relations with others. This is, of course, part and parcel of the genre of autobiography: it is not that de Beauvoir is the only author who writes in this way. But it is the case that de Beauvoir's very comprehensiveness, the sheer extent of the autobiography, invites expectations of revelation and 'knowing all'. As it is, we learn a great deal about the texture of her life, since de Beauvoir

provides rich and detailed accounts of her childhood, adolescence and maturity, but rather less about the person within this
texture. Yet this is still to linger with the expectation that a person
writing an autobiography will reveal themselves explicitly and
offer an account which includes as much of their negative selves
as the more positive aspects. What is tantalising about de Beauvoir is her apparent promise of revelation. As readers we are
invited to believe that her autobiography will tell us about her. As
written, it certainly fulfils the promise of telling us a great deal
about de Beauvoir, yet at the same time we are not trusted, as
readers, with anything other than the most morally positive
account of de Beauvoir's actions. Thus we are presented with an
extremely Catholic version of a life: a life justified and legitimated
through individual acts in which we are strongly encouraged to
endorse the actor.

Yet this explicitly Catholic form of moral legitimacy collapses
in the face of the crisis provoked in de Beauvoir's life by the death
of her mother, which is discussed in *A Very Easy Death*.[26] This slim
volume covers a relatively short period in de Beauvoir's life, the
months between the onset of debility in Françoise de Beauvoir
and her death from cancer. The most striking aspect of the work
is de Beauvoir's reaction to the death of her mother :

> Why did my mother's death shake me so deeply? Since the
> time I left home I had felt little in the way of emotional
> impulse towards her . . . Generally speaking I thought of her
> with no particular feeling. Yet in my sleep (although my
> father only made very rare and then insignificant appear-
> ances) she often played a most important part: she blended
> with Sartre, and we were happy together. And then the
> dream would turn into a nightmare: why was I living with
> her once more? How had I come to be in her power again?
> So our former relationship lived on in me in its double aspect
> – a subjection that I loved and hated.[27]

The passage illustrates, in the most perfect, textbook form that duality of feeling about mothers which Melanie Klein identified. De Beauvoir's positive and happy feeling about her mother, and her physical delight at her mother in childhood and infancy are very evident in *Memoirs of a Dutiful Daughter*. The book is almost elegiac in its treatment of the sumptuous delights, the delicious food, the oral gratification provided by those early years. Then, as readers know, poverty and a harsh reality set in. The mother is no longer the delightful warm person who feeds and provides intense feeling of pleasure; she becomes instead the person who threatens de Beauvoir's autonomy and sense of self. The text follows all those aspects of mother love/mother hatred which Klein outlined: the pleasure mixed with the fear and the seeking for external means of resolving what appears to be the chaos threatened by the mother. As Janet Sayers points out, in her account of Melanie Klein:

> Furthermore, she [Melanie Klein] argued that through schoolwork the child seeks to reassure itself that it has the inner capacity to make good any harm done the loved mother by envy and hatred of her. Similar motives, she said, impel the search of adults for sexual approval and sex, and women's child-bearing, breast-feeding and caring activity generally. Where all goes well such activity serves to convince us of our capacity to make good any harm done to self or others by the hatred and envy first felt toward the mother.[28]

Readers of de Beauvoir would probably find it impossible to find in de Beauvoir's autobiography much evidence of her desire to replicate the caring, maternal functions of her mother. On the other hand, evidence could be found in considerable quantities about reassurance by academic work and sexual encounters. Of both of these forms of emotional order, the autobiography gives ample instances.

Nevertheless, what de Beauvoir gives us in *Memoirs of a Dutiful Daughter* is a rational, and rationalising, account of her scholastic commitment. For her, the energy she devoted to her studies has nothing to do for a search for inner coherence but everything to do with a desire for coherence in the world, and for control in it. The fusion in the de Beauvoir household of the ordinary pattern of love/hate between children and their mothers thus took place against a particularly fertile background in which the ordinary contradictions of psycho-sexual family relationships were worked out in a way which integrated irrational needs with those of the rational world. De Beauvoir, just like millions of other human beings, needed to resolve her contradictory and ambivalent feelings about her mother. Equally, she needed to provide for herself and to provide for herself in such a way as to allow her to remain securely located within the bourgeoisie. Thus, at the same time as providing, through academic success, a way of defining herself and bringing coherence to her world, this commitment allowed her two advantages: the promise of future personal autonomy, and a rational account of the world which appeared to put herself at a safe distance from the religious knowledge and understanding of her mother. The secular religion of the rational placed de Beauvoir firmly with her father; an identification which again had dual advantages – resolution and affirmation in the emotional world and a means of securing an independent self in reality.

Given the possible rewards of academic dedication, it is little wonder that the adolescent Simone gave her complete attention to examination success. Although she occasionally includes disclaimers about her dedication ('All the time I was trying so hard not be a little book-worm'), the thread of *Memoirs of a Dutiful Daughter* is one which leads inexorably from the confusions of childhood to the resolution of scholastic success.[29] With furious energy, de Beauvoir devotes herself to working herself out of the ambiguities of family and home: part of this process of emancipation includes the beginning of the relationship with Sartre, and the start of a partnership which was to become part of the mythology of European intellectual life.

By the time that de Beauvoir embarked on her autobiographical project, she and Sartre were established as well-known figures of the European political and intellectual circles. Their names had become closely linked, and it was commonplace to regard their relationship as something close to conventional marriage. *Memoirs of a Dutiful Daughter* was published in 1958, and the other volumes of autobiography followed: *The Prime of Life* (1960), *Force of Circumstance* (1963) and *All Said and Done* (1972). When she began to write *Memoirs*, de Beauvoir was forty-eight years old, and of her decision to abandon fiction for autobiography, her biographer Deirdre Bair says:

> In 1957, as she began to write her autobiography, she had just ended fifteen years of concentrating upon herself in her writing, but always from the distance required by the particular form of the work. Now she decided to address her situation head on, without the buffers of various conventions of genre.[30]

The question that de Beauvoir set out to answer in her autobiography was, Bair writes, a question de Beauvoir herself posed: 'My life: it is both intimately known and remote: it defines me and yet I stand outside it. Just what, precisely, is this curious object?'[31] The question radiates that idea of distinct and separate selves; Bair's view is that de Beauvoir's autobiography provides a 'generally scrupulously honest self-examination'.[32]

This optimistic, and sympathetic account of de Beauvoir's autobiography is one which is perhaps inevitable, given the close relationship between Bair and de Beauvoir to the subject of de Beauvoir. Biographies are sometimes described as definitive, or authorised, or critical; the biography of de Beauvoir by Bair might well be described as a partnership between subject and author. There can be little doubt of the part de Beauvoir played in the biography; at many points in Bair's narrative, de Beauvoir's voice interjects to impose or offer her account of events. Bair makes no secret of the way she worked on the construction of the manuscript of the biography with de Beauvoir, nor does she conceal her view that de Beauvoir's work, in particular *The Second Sex*, was 'largely responsible (in my mind at least) for many

of the opportunities that were available to women of my generation.'[33] This view, echoed by the quotation at the end of the
biography in which Elisabeth Badinter is cited as saying 'Women,
you owe everything to her!', is part of the mythology which sur-
rounds de Beauvoir, and which, of course, she went some way to
construct.

Thus alternative views of de Beauvoir's autobiography can
take issue not just with the degree of accuracy – on a purely
factual level – of the work, but also with the contribution made
by the author to the emancipation of women. What is now
regarded within feminism as 'standpoint' theory, suggests that
it is impossible to study or record the world without some
declaration of the position of the person who is the author of the
record.[34] The idea was formulated to challenge the claims of
'objectivity' in the human and natural sciences, claims which
frequently marginalised or obscured the interests of women. In
de Beauvoir's autobiography (and indeed in her pivotal work on
women, *The Second Sex*), it is apparent that the relationship
between de Beauvoir *and* women and de Beauvoir *as* woman is an
intensely problematic one. Throughout her autobiography, and
throughout *The Second Sex*, de Beauvoir locates herself as the
observer and the commentator on the position of women;
women are 'they', and from the beginning to the conclusion of
the book, the author's stand is one of dispassionate observation.
This does not mean that de Beauvoir is not passionate about the
position of women, and often clearly enraged by aspects of misogyny in Western culture, but there is a distance, and a separation, which is inescapable. It is all the more ironic that this sense
of distance is so much a part of de Beauvoir, given that the
analysis provided by de Beauvoir is so dichotomous; women and
men being two essentially separate categories. Radical feminists
such as Kate Millett and Shulamith Firestone had no difficulty
in identifying with de Beauvoir, indeed Firestone's *The Dialectic of
Sex* is dedicated to Simone de Beauvoir. But at the same time
as this identification makes absolute sense of the perception of
difference between women and men that is a part of radical

feminism, it also ignores the way in which de Beauvoir seeks the resolution of women's subordination in identity with masculinity.

To say this of the woman regarded as the 'mother' of European feminism clearly has heretical possibilities. But what the identity, and sense of identity is about, is identification with masculinity in an abstract form – the intellectual power and competence, and the possibility of a transcendent intelligence which de Beauvoir locates in men rather than women. It is not, it must be emphasised, that de Beauvoir is arguing that men are more intelligent or more capable of abstract thought than women, but that the condition of masculinity – its lack, in particular, of subjectivity – makes it the definitive condition of intellectual life. Given that de Beauvoir's sense of values and aspiration is located firmly within the intellectual world, it is hardly surprising that her standards are firmly placed within masculinity. So, too, is the subject matter of her autobiography: the public world is represented by engagement in national and international politics, the private world (certainly not absent in de Beauvoir) by a discussion of the state of her relationship with Sartre and significant other men. The death of her mother is compartmentalised into a separate volume. Women, this implicit separation seems to be suggesting, are not part of the narrative project of post-Enlightenment rationality.

Yet of course de Beauvoir, as her childhood heroines indicate, was desperate to be the person who controlled and directed her own narrative. But, as her reading of fiction in adolescence indicated, there are few women in fiction who achieve heroic status. Women became tragic heroines, but in the nineteenth- and twentieth-century literature which de Beauvoir knew, there were few women who achieved personal autonomy of a genuinely heroic kind. Little wonder, then, that in writing her autobiography de Beauvoir set out to write for herself a narrative of heroic achievement. She does not separate herself from the child and the adolescent: her objectives in life are stated in *Memoirs of a Dutiful Daughter* and the theme of life as a project, the definitive organising purpose of masculine modernity dominates the four volumes of autobiography. There are inevitably ups and downs on the way, and to de Beauvoir's intense (and very honest) amazement other people intervene in her life in ways which she had not expected. (Most dramatically, for example, in 1940 the Germans invade Paris.) Sartre is a constant source of concern and anxiety; in the early years of the relationship the problems are concentrated around his relations with other women, in later life the problems became those of his health and his collapse into debility and dependence. Nevertheless, despite these numerous problems, de Beauvoir continues with an optimistic vision of the possibilities of her life. In her sixties and seventies she is prepared to take on new intellectual challenges, enter new relationships and continue to engage with European politics.

This endless vitality can be attributed to a number of factors in de Beauvoir's life. By all accounts, her mother passed on to de Beauvoir a sense of constant interest in the world and events; as in many mother/daughter relationships, the unresolved ambiguities of the relationship gave both parties a sense of energy and engagement. Equally, de Beauvoir had, in Sartre, a figure around whom she could organise her intellectual and imaginative life, and yet one on whom she did not have to depend for day-to-day support. When Sartre's health did decline, it is clear that the convention of separate households was one that was of enormous advantage to de Beauvoir, as were the young women who were willing to provide domestic aid for Sartre. Thus the function of Sartre as a location of intellectual imagination was enormously significant, but not one that in de Beauvoir's case carried the usual and conventional costs of domestic care. But the cost of Sartre as an object of phallic identity and order was the imprisoning of de Beauvoir within the specifics of the totalising, systematic nature of Sartre's own intellectual project. Few readers of *The Prime of Life* can escape the impression that what Sartre possessed was a very considerable sense of grandiosity: he wished to produce a definitive philosophical system and had little doubt of his ability to do this. Whether or not he actually did this was, however, becoming something of a redundant question after

1945, in that, while Sartre and de Beauvoir were locked into their projects of providing comprehensive and definitive explanations of moral action and the situation of women, the world changed, and the importance of these projects changed.

If de Beauvoir's autobiography therefore leaves much excluded, in that she very clearly and deliberately leaves out many aspects of her relationships with others, particularly female others, it is equally a monumental work of traditional narrative. It is impossible not to observe that de Beauvoir simply refuses a discussion of her bisexuality and her sexual relations with women. To the end of her life, she refused all attempts to define her sexuality in terms which might have included women as well. Clearly, the symbolic costs of this possibility were too considerable, and too considerably negative, for de Beauvoir. Thus, as much as the distortions which sometimes appear in de Beauvoir's autobiography, we also have to name the numerous absences – and high among those absences are two kinds of human relationships: sexual relations between women, and fleeting heterosexual relations. The picture which de Beauvoir paints of herself in her autobiography is thus of a woman who had three significant sexual relationships with men: Sartre, Algren and Lanzmann. Other lovers are not mentioned. This exclusion could have many perfectly justifiable explanations, but one explanation deserves mention: that de Beauvoir wished to portray herself as different from Sartre in her sexual relations with others and was still sufficiently part of her bourgeois background to be wary of what she once described as 'promiscuity' in women.

This explanation of an individual's perception of manners and morality is one which may be responsible for de Beauvoir's absence of revelation in her autobiography. Another possibility is that she was so concerned with the construction of herself as the heroine of her own narrative, that she did not wish to admit those aspects of her own behaviour which might not have accorded with her interpretation of this project. In writing her autobiography de Beauvoir knew full well that autobiographies (let alone four-volume autobiographies) by women are relatively rare, and that, as a woman famous before the publication of her autobiography, hers would inevitably attract attention. To make herself a legend in her lifetime would not fit easily with accounts of relationships founded in less than appropriately serious needs and desires. Equally, de Beauvoir's perception of sexuality was always one which involved an uneasy mix of heterosexual conquest, voyeurism and competition. For the French historian of sexuality Michel Foucault, de Beauvoir was a source of constant irritation and dislike: here was a woman endorsing the emancipation of women and yet apparently deeply tied to phallic primacy.[35] Since Foucault's own theoretical energies were all directed towards separating sexuality, and sexual pleasure, from the burdens of morality, accounts of the world such as de Beauvoir's were inevitably distant and hostile.

Yet in the latter part of the twentieth century it was the influence of Foucault that became central to Western interpretations of sexuality. What we can note, however, is that in de Beauvoir's autobiography, and her account of post-war intellectual life in France, Foucault does not appear. Hence, at the same time as de Beauvoir avoids all mention of those personal relationships which might undermine her sense of herself, so she avoids all intellectual figures who represent significant challenges. Foremost among twentieth-century figures of this kind is Freud, but a long list of other absent figures can be gathered. With the challenges that these figures represent to the content of de Beauvoir's work goes another, equally serious challenge. It is that of suggesting a different position in relationship to knowledge to that of de Beauvoir, a position which does not attempt totality, allows subjectivity and has abandoned the idea of heroism and the intact subject. In short, it is a way of looking at the world which is the inevitable result of modernity and post-modernity. The definitive self – that central belief of the nineteenth-century bourgeoisie – was constructed around the separation of the world into the public and the private and the location of agency in the male public world. To be female was to be excluded from agency, and the history of the nineteenth and twentieth centuries is replete with instances of the struggles of women (and men) to renegotiate this paralysing division. Yet, as much as the male, active self was the ideal form of nineteenth-century bourgeois society, so it was an endlessly problematic self: the rigid hero of bourgeois society was shown, in novels, autobiography and the sheer evidence of everyday life, to be a weak and hapless figure. The sexual reformers of late Victorian England, and the increasingly public homosexual voice, ruthlessly derided this absurd figure. In England, the actual people of Bloomsbury, as well as their works, seriously undermined conventional expectations of masculinity. Traditional, rugged masculinity had its literary defenders in writers such as D.H. Lawrence, but in the main the twentieth-century direction of fiction (not to mention everyday life) was towards a more diverse and diffuse masculinity.

None of this sense of diversity, and the deconstruction of masculinity is apparent in de Beauvoir. Men are, and largely remain, heroes, and they are such because of their intellectual agency. (It is notable that few homosexual figures appear in de Beauvoir; when they do they are presented as unhappy and unsuccessful people.) This places women in a situation that is a poor fit with both reality and the intellectual possibilities of the twentieth century. Women's lives generally move between the public and the private; equally, the crucial feature of modernity has, from the late nineteenth century, been its understanding and inclusion of femininity. Thus the misogynist male writers who appear in *The Second Sex* do not represent twentieth-century literature *per se*, so much as a reaction to the threat in twentieth-century literature of the symbolic presence of femininity and the literal presence of women. What we are given, therefore, both in de Beauvoir's autobiography and *The Second Sex*, is an account of gender relations that is essentially located within a nineteenth-century model of masculine heroism. Within this model, de Beauvoir is to be a hero; she succeeds in becoming a model of the possibilities of female agency, but a model that is deeply and crucially dependent upon a fantasy of masculinity. In order to achieve her own heroism, de Beauvoir had to continue to invent, and invest in, masculinity. What her autobiography offers to us, therefore, is a superbly articulate instance of the possibilities of the invention of the other – but in this case, an other who never existed in reality and was rapidly being challenged theoretically. 'If God did not exist, we should have to invent him' is a remark from another context which suggests much of the intensely fictional quality of de Beauvoir's autobiography, an autobiography in which the mass of descriptive detail about the life of a woman cannot entirely obscure the ever-present, and ever-powerful, generalised male other.

Chapter 3

Imperatives of deference

To construct a fantasy about oneself is hardly an unusual human act, even if few of us go to the same lengths as Simone de Beauvoir to ensure that we exercise the maximum degree of control over our created selves. Equally common, if more socially significant, is the creation and continuation through auto/biography of fantasies about others. A particular instance of these created fantasies are auto/biographies about the British Royal Family – auto/biographies that have played a part in maintaining the reverence of the monarchy which is only now beginning to disappear. On the library shelves of autobiography and biography, the British Royal Family occupies a not inconsiderable space. The very longevity of the English, and subsequently the British, Royal Family gives biographers considerable scope. There are almost no figures in the history of English and British royalty who do not have their biographer: from Alfred the Great to Elizabeth II, the figures are the subjects of tirelessly researched and richly detailed accounts of their lives. But over many of the figures, and certainly the figures from Queen Victoria onwards, there hangs a curtain of discretion and often sheer evasion. Given that the British Royal Family is precisely that – a family – one of the major evasions in writing about it is the refusal of most biographers to consider it as such, and to remark on the quite considerable continuities within it. In the light of recent events surrounding the British Royal Family, these continuities demand mention, as does the extraordinary ability of the British royal family to continue in a century which has not been generally sympathetic to monarchies.

Yet in this context, we also have to say that no century, and no place, is particularly sympathetic to monarchies. 'Uneasy lies the head that wears a crown', fairly adequately sums up the perils of being a monarch. Equally – given the conduct of many monarchs – an uneasy rest is perfectly justifiable. Given that the behaviour has often been appalling, there has never been any reason to condone it. Nevertheless, European societies have been monarch-prone and, for reasons that have yet to be adequately explained, have shown a continued propensity to endorse their national identity with a monarch. The making (literally) of kingdoms has generally involved a king, and these kings have become the rallying-points for national identity. At certain points in British history, most notably the eighteenth century, the extreme incapacity (not to mention foreign birth) of monarchs might have coincided with a rejection of the British monarchy, yet the very incompetence of the crown seems, in a paradoxical way, to have made the institution of monarchy in Britain stronger. Precisely because successive Hanoverian Georges were so notably disinclined to rule, in anything like the same sense as monarchs elsewhere, they became more important as symbolic representations of nationhood. The fantasy of the monarch thus became far more effective than the reality.

This disjunction between fantasy and reality was, perhaps unfortunately for the long-term prospects of the House of Windsor, systematically and deliberately closed in the reign of Queen Victoria. The Queen, and still more her German consort, Prince Albert, did not choose to go on living their lives in whatever kind of personal disarray they found most appropriate. Instead they wished to 'set an example' and separate themselves as rapidly and thoroughly as possible from the dissolute behaviour of Victoria's uncles. The young queen acted with personal generosity and lack of animosity towards the scattered and often penniless remnants of George III's family, but she made it absolutely clear that she did not wish to choose or condone the same kind of private life for herself. Indeed, within ten years of her accession, Victoria and Albert had made it plain that they wished to bring together the reality of the personal behaviour of the monarch (and in this case her family) with expectations of absolute adherence to certain kinds of moral standards. Central to these standards was a belief in fidelity in marriage for both parties (an idea which was to prove calamitous for the Windsors in the twentieth century) and a commitment to royal duty above and beyond personal inclination and need. Victoria and Albert, in order to establish the kind of moral dynasty which they saw as appropriate, instituted the kind of particularly brutal training of the eldest son which was to prove such a fateful decision.

The rigorous training of the future Edward VII was, as some contemporary observers pointed out, both cruel and ineffective.[1] 'Bertie' had no especial intellectual gifts and more strikingly – although far less often observed either by his parents or subsequent biographers – entirely ordinary needs for affection, support and reward. Given that he could not meet the obsessive standards of his father, poor Bertie became a disappointment to his parents and an indirect cause, according to his mother, of his father's death. It is a great tribute to the capacity of Edward VII to seek pleasure that, despite the black gloom that descended on his mother after Albert's death (and to a certain extent the work-crazy gloom within which Albert lived), he continued to seek sensual gratification until the time of his death. 'Edwardian' became a code word for hedonism, the escape and evasion from Victorian values, particularly in terms of sexual morality. The wealth that a tiny section of the Edwardian population enjoyed allowed both absolute exclusion from any mundane demands, while increasingly democratic ideas and practices marginalised the direct political influence of the throne. Towards the end of her life, Victoria was held in considerable public esteem. After the strains inflicted on the monarchy by Victoria's virtual seclusion after Albert's death, both mother and son lived to see the triumphant entry of the British monarchy into the twentieth century. The family had been saved from a potentially disastrous succession by the death of the eldest son of Edward VII and Princess Alexandra. Writing in 1982 of the death of the inadequate Prince Albert Victor, Elizabeth Longford noted discreetly that Prince George (the future George V) 'possessed qualities conspicuously lacking in his brother'.[2]

Prince Eddy's 'inadequacy' lay in what seems to have been a real difficulty with any kind of educational achievement as much as his refusal to embrace the public heterosexuality and rugged masculinity which was then expected of British upper-class men. With the engaging frankness and absolute ruthlessness of judgement of which she was often capable, Queen Victoria noted, on Eddy's death, that it was not altogether an unhappy event. She mourned for his parents, but it is apparent that she could not entirely mourn for the country. Always a realist, she was worldly enough to recognise that whatever Eddy's personal life was like, his real problem was his lack of intelligence. Even if his father was hardly academically gifted, he was shrewd enough in his judgements and assessments of the world.

The monarchy which entered the twentieth century was thus one which had been recast, in the nineteenth century, in terms of identity with particular kinds of moral values and personal behaviour. It was a behaviour based on heterosexual marriage and committed to a division of the sexes which rigidly compartmentalised behaviour, inclination and attitude into 'feminine' and 'masculine'. Women were expected to be chaste before marriage and accept male infidelity as part and parcel of the conventions of marriage. Queen Victoria and Prince Albert were both fervent in their condemnation of this double standard in sexual behaviour and attempted to impress their children and their court with this expectation. It was to the lasting disadvantage of the British monarchy that they succeeded in neither endeavour: they failed to change the practice of aristocratic sexual licence which had always tolerated properly managed and arranged infidelity within marriage, and they failed to prevent their sons from internalising these expectations. Edward VII, in the words of his biographers, 'enjoyed' the company of numerous women other than his wife whilst his son, the supposedly respectable George V, rejoiced prior to his marriage in the company of a woman he described as a 'little ripper'.[3]

What biographers have done with this pattern of behaviour has been to apply a degree of literary lip-service to the idea of regret from the departure from conventional morality. At the same time, from the pages of Philip Magnus on Edward VII and Kenneth Rose on George V, it is apparent that the 'little ripper' and the royal mistresses of Edward VII are acceptable because they did not threaten the monarchy in any way, and above all accepted the rules and conventions which governed bourgeois and aristocratic social and personal life. Those surrounding the monarchy observed discretion, the parties concerned 'knew their place' and the codes of dress, etiquette, appearance and behaviour were all observed. It is apparent from his justifications of Edward VII's liaisons that Philip Magnus recognised the potential hurt to Queen Alexandra of these relationships, but the king is excused on the grounds that Queen Alexandra (owing to her hearing problems) could not enjoy society, and that whatever he did, the king was always meticulous in observing strict codes of etiquette.[4] In this biography there is clearly a sense that the king did not always behave quite like an English gentleman, but Magnus cannot find either the nerve or the heart to censor him. Aside from this failure of moral will, Magnus also did not have at his command a language or an understanding to explain Edward VII's behaviour or to see it in terms of the long-term credibility of the monarch.

The biography of Edward VII by Philip Magnus was one of the first post-Second World War biographies to turn to a discussion of the Royal Family. As such, the biographer had to deal with a culture and a country which was largely innocent of the possibility of hostility to the Royal Family. This is not to say that there was not a considerable degree of latent republicanism, in the sense that many people had little respect for the Royal Family and even less toleration for its vast privilege. But this strand of distance from the Royal Family seldom hardened into explicit calls for the abolition of the monarchy. By the time Kenneth Rose published his account of the life of George V (in 1983), the monarchy could still call on considerable public support, but thinking about morality and sexuality – crucial areas in any discussion about the monarchy – had changed. The understanding of gender relations had been sharpened by feminism, and the shifts in public morality identified as part of the 'permissive' society had made the codes of aristocratic sexuality appear both hypocritical and misogynist. Thus, even though Kenneth Rose was clearly writing very firmly, and very clearly, within a proroyalist framework (the biography is dedicated to 'Edward, Duke of Kent, grandson of King George V'), he could comment on the 'humiliation' experienced by Queen Alexandra as a result of her husband's relations with other women, and assess the relations of Edward VII and the future George V in terms of a wider understanding of the social world:

> The Prince of Wales displayed not only the understandable loyalty of a son to his father, but also the awe of a subject for his sovereign. That one king at least could do no wrong was for him not so much a constitutional dictum as a literal truth. He took a hierarchical view of humanity: the rich king in his castle, the rich prince at his gate. While his father lived, this subservience robbed their intimacy of spontaneity and vigour; and once Prince George had himself succeeded to the throne, it inhibited his own relationship with both wife and children.[5]

Rose, throughout his five hundred pages about George V, remains intensely loyal to his subject, but he cannot avoid discourses about politics and emotional life which by the 1970s and 1980s had begun to invade even the circles of royal biographers. Furthermore, he was writing after the publication in 1974 of Frances Donaldson's biography of Edward VIII, a biography that made absolutely apparent (as did Philip Ziegler's later biography of the same subject) Edward's problematic and difficult relationships with women.[6] Rose acknowledges Edward VIII's long-standing affair with Mrs Dudley Ward, and makes no secret of the fact that the only women to whom Edward VIII was attracted were married. Yet at the same time, Rose goes to some lengths to assert that Edward VIII (like his brothers and sisters) had a happy childhood, was kindly treated and enjoyed friendly relations with his parents. The manifest evidence within the family of emotional disturbance (George VI's stutter, for example, and Edward VIII's attraction to married women) is passed over in the same way that Queen Mary's behaviour as a mother (or lack of behaviour as a mother) is defended.

Yet just one year before Rose's biography of George V, a biographer of his son, George VI, had written on the same subject of royal parent/child relations:

> The future Queen Mary was prey to acute shyness and so reserved in her emotions that she found it almost impossible to express them freely to her small children. The Empress Frederick considered her to be 'very cold and stiff and very unmaternal'. According to Frances Donaldson, 'Someone who knew her in later life summed up what dozens of people bear witness to by saying: "Queen Mary had nothing of the mother at all."' So crippling was her inability to communicate easily with others, at least during this early stage of her marriage, that it was left to her husband to rebuke servants or alter arrangements for the children. Between her young children and her there was a chilling distance, and it is significant that she once wrote to her husband of her eldest son: 'I really believe he begins to like me at last, he is most civil to me.' Later, 'I have always to remember that their father is also their King.'[7]

Judd (the author of the passage above), Donaldson and Ziegler now represent the consensus of royal biographers that, whatever the good intentions, the home life of the British Royal Family in

the twentieth century has been very far from happy. No biographer has suggested deliberate malice or cruelty on the part of
any royal parent (although royal nannies seem to be rather different), but it is apparent, and publicly apparent, that the people
who emerged from these royal nurseries had considerable
difficulty in relating to others.

But in making these comments, a number of observations also
have to be made. First, the assumptions of close ties between
parents (particularly mothers) and children is a relatively modern
one and dates, at least in theoretical terms, from the work in the
1930s and 1940s of Anna Freud, D.W. Winnicott and John
Bowlby on maternal deprivation. The centrality of the mother in
the child's early life has become an assumption of the late twentieth century, but no such idea existed to protect the royal children from the habits that assumed that infants and children could
be cared for in ways which separated them from both their physical mothers and their surrogates. Thus we might explain the
behaviour of Queen Mary by reference to the standards of aristocratic child-rearing of the time. More telling, and in many ways
more problematic, was the childhood constructed for Prince
Charles, George VI's grandson. The image of the five-year-old
prince shaking hands on meeting his mother suggests a considerable degree of difference from patterns which by that time, the
early 1950s, had become generalised. The separation of child
and parents endlessly engaged in by wealthy families was part
and parcel of this family experience; in the guise of a determination to allow the heir to the throne an 'ordinary' childhood, a
degree of separation was established which was absolutely not
ordinary and was becoming less common even for the most
wealthy.

The 'Windsors trample on their young' is a well-known remark
about the British Royal Family, and any reading of royal biography in the twentieth century must confirm lives of misery and
unhappiness lived in conditions of wealth and privilege. Edward
VIII escaped this world by marriage to the second great
dominatrix of his life, Mrs Simpson. George VI passed on to his

daughters a crippling sense of duty which was later to disable many of his grandchildren. Thus the second point to consider here is the nature of the imperative which made this behaviour apparently necessary. Edward VII had recognised that a large part of his popularity lay in his very failings: his enthusiasms for eating, horse-racing and women largely endeared him to his subjects, and there was little overt criticism of his consistent sexual deviance. But at the same time, the standards of the time tolerated distinctions between public and private, and endorsed the breaking of rules in rule-bound ways. The tragedy for George V and his descendants was that modernity had so such toleration: public and private boundaries were eroded, rules were questioned and discourses of sexuality were challenged in ways that made conventional constructions of masculinity and femininity more problematic. Thus, while both Edward VII and George V attached enormous importance to dress, since in doing so they literally as well as symbolically 'put on' kingship, Edward VIII flouted existing expectations about dressing. When the royal body was finally exposed (in the shape of Edward VIII in bathing clothes when on holiday with Mrs Simpson), a line was crossed in which reality finally challenged the imagination. Here, at last, was a man, and a rather small and physically frail man at that. In a decade in which ideas about masculinity were being extended and contested by a generation that included the politically radical and openly homosexual writers Auden and Isherwood, the literal recognition of the King as Man inevitably brought home to many subjects the possibility of considering the limits of deference.

From the time of the Abdication, the British monarchy thus had to be remade. The king, whether Edward VIII or George VI, was in no sense a model of manhood and masculinity, and by this point it was apparent that an increasingly self-confident mass media (derived initially from the more socially democratic United States), were not likely to allow distance between king and subjects to remain. The literal and the symbolic somehow had to be reunited. With the exquisite absence of social understanding that has often characterised their dealings with the wider world, the House of Windsor chose the patriarchal nuclear family as their pivotal identification. Victoria and Albert had made their personal stance one of opposition to what they perceived as the dissolute behaviour of their various relatives. As many biographers of Queen Victoria have pointed out, the crucial figure in this campaign was not so much the Queen (with whose name all things repressive are, often quite falsely, associated) as Prince Albert. Dorothy Thompson wrote of Albert:

> He was in many ways a quite exceptional character to find among the royal personages of Europe. He was able, conscientious, moderately religious, a devoted family man, a good administrator and a competent behind the scenes operator. In the early years of the reign when the queen was very much occupied with producing children, his support and guidance became absolutely essential to her.[8]

The crucial sentence here is 'a quite exceptional character to find among the royal personages of Europe', since what Thompson recognises, more clearly and explicitly than many other writers of royal biographies, is that if ever talent, competence and moral continence were absent in human beings, this was often the case among monarchs. These were 'missing persons' in a quite literal sense, in that, far from simply failing to measure up to the absurd and inflated expectations of kingship, they equally failed to meet the standards and expectations of most of their subjects. With his enthusiasms for education and science, and his learned expertise in the ways of mid-nineteenth-century diplomacy, Albert offered a reality of competence to the British monarchy which has never, in modern years, been surpassed. Indeed, what he managed to do was to perform a lesson in democracy that was particularly fitting in the age of parliamentary reform and the extension of higher education, fulfilling many of the expectations of educated middle-class men in Victorian England.

But these ordinary, human talents were not passed on to subsequent monarchs. Albert's eldest daughter (who became the Empress of Prussia) was a clever and liberal woman, but the impact of her gender, particularly at the repressive and illiberal Prussian court, was considerable. As the throne passed to Edward VII, George V and briefly to Edward VIII, it passed to men who could take on only a rigid model of their given role in order to achieve any credibility. The testimony of tutors, teachers and contemporaries of all these men attests to their intellectual impoverishment, their emotional under-development and their rigid, and often obsessive, concern with matters of form and dress. By 1936 and the time of the Abdication, it was apparent that the House of Windsor could produce a certain kind of man, one who might become respected if – and only if – he obeyed to the letter the forms and expectations of kingship. In an age in which hedonism and personal fulfilment became part of the dominating social ethos, Edward VIII was unable to match his democratic aspirations to expectations of him as a king. The crisis provoked by the romantic entanglement of this supremely troubled monarch was both a personal and a general crisis for the Windsors: the identity of the monarchy had been organised around strict codes of sexual behaviour, particularly by George V. Given this identification (an identification which refused any toleration of divorced people and provoked George V's remark about a homosexual that 'I always thought that people like that shot themselves'), the Windsors were left with little space in which to negotiate changes and shifts in the monarchy.[9]

In the years after the Abdication, the problems of Edward VIII could be explained as single phenomenon in an otherwise unbroken line of royal good behaviour and acceptable competence. Writing about Edward VIII as a moral incompetent and personally inadequate human being did not take great effort; the evidence was considerable, and there have clearly been many close to the Royal Family who were happy to collude with the demonisation of the man who so flagrantly rejected many of the values for which the British Establishment stood. Making

Edward VIII into a hopeless and hapless case thus had a real political significance to it. Thankfully, the forces of stability could argue, this man was just exceptionally weak, and luckily there was a younger brother who was regarded as perfect for the role of king. This legitimation excuses from blame the parents, the court and the social world that produced Edward VIII and evades discussion of the issue of the monarchy's determination to maintain, at whatever cost, the institution of a hereditary throne. In reading both Frances Donaldson and Philip Ziegler on Edward VIII, it is apparent that a very large number of people were involved in ensuring that the monarchy continued, and moreover continued in the way which they thought suitable. The meaning of this suitability was fixed in terms that were completely literal and were subsequently to prove disastrous for a later generation. But the literal meaning decided for the monarchy in the 1930s was that the monarch should embody the expectations of bourgeois family life within the context of aristocratic privilege. The inevitable tensions and contradictions set up by this *concordat* were not at first apparent: George VI and Queen Elizabeth actually lived the respectable family life that was expected of them and passed on to their eldest daughter an absolute veneration for the institution of monarchy. Thus in these persons what was deemed suitable actually coincided with the personalities and the circumstances of the individuals concerned. The conditions of the Second World War allowed the monarchy a degree of identification with its subjects, and the gender of the sovereign's children made them less vulnerable to the brutalising socialisation into masculinity that had been the fate of Edward VII, George V, Edward VIII and George VI.

But the process of brutalisation was again returned to in the education of Prince Charles. Despite a culture which was, by the 1950s, beginning to recognise the emotional fragility of children, Prince Charles was exposed to the terrors of an early separation from home and the deprivations of a particularly harsh boarding school.[10] This process was yet again conducted in terms of that double imperative which had made miserable the childhoods of previous monarchs. First, the king-to-be must learn the accepted pattern of conventional masculinity which excludes affectivity (not to mention the company of women). Second, the king-to-be must learn to mix with 'ordinary' children and youths. The non-sense of this idea has always been transparent, since no king-to-be has ever experienced the education of the majority of his subjects. The dialectic of ordinary and privileged thus dominated the education of Prince Charles in the same way as for previous generations, and in the same way it failed in both respects, being neither 'ordinary' in the sense of shared, nor 'privileged' in the sense of allowing any space for individual inclination or taste.

What the education did was, predictably, produce the kind of person typical of Windsor males, a person dominated by a set of imperatives imposed by others. Brought up in a household of some formality and endlessly told of his 'difference' from others, it was inevitable that what should emerge was a person entirely similar to the most unfortunate of his subjects – similar in the very sense that most of his 'ordinary' needs and desires had been ruthlessly denied. All this was, of course, accomplished in the light of an assumption that no alternative was possible. The imperatives were not, then, of an individual's own making but derived from the sense of those surrounding him that any departure from known patterns would be dangerous and damaging. As a family the Windsors, particularly its female members, have a quite explicit wish to maintain their powers and privilege. Ziegler's biography of Edward VIII makes plain, for example, the ruthless determination of Queen Elizabeth, the Queen Mother, to isolate Edward VIII and his wife from anything to do with the monarchy.[11] The same person was equally prepared to ensure that their younger daughter relinquished her chosen marriage, on the grounds that the husband-to-be was divorced. In this there is, of course, a terrible irony, in that just at the time when Princess Margaret gave up the idea of marriage to Peter Townsend, divorce became increasingly common among her sister's subjects and was to become a more than common experience among her immediate family.

The working out of the drama of Windsors thus shows certain continuities, all of them yielding disastrous results for the individuals concerned. The male members of the family have been subjected to a ruthless socialisation which effectively limits their human capacities, while the family itself both chooses and is ruled by attitudes and social relationships largely different and distinct from the majority of the population. In this it is important to emphasise the limits of the agency of the Royal Family; one interpretation of the Saga of Windsor is that of a family freely choosing and directing its fate, but to ascribe this degree of active direction to the family is misleading. From the time of Queen Victoria onwards, it is apparent that the monarch had a portion of great privilege (in the material sense) but was also deeply circumscribed by a hierarchical court system. Queen Victoria and Prince Albert established an ethos of anti-luxury at court, and Queen Victoria (very much like King George V and King George VI) was fond of proclaiming to the world her enthusiasm for the simple life. To this end, all three monarchs subjected their family and their courtiers to various kinds of physical rigour, ranging from the freezing cold enjoyed by Queen Victoria in her residences to the deliberate deprivations forced on their children by George V and to a lesser extent Edward VII. (Again, the children of George VI, being girls, largely escaped this pattern.) This deliberate choice of hardship and the non-luxurious was then justified in terms of the very 'ordinary' habits of the monarch. To have delighted in luxury, ostentation and pleasure would have been out of step with the perceived values of the monarchy's subjects.

Yet from all the biographical material now available about the British Royal Family, it is apparent that the individual members have had little or no immediate experience of what passes for everyday experience for the majority of their citizens. The physical isolation of the Royal Family ensures that travel and movement are always segregated. Their vast wealth ensures that choices about material life seldom have to be made, and the numbers of the support staff make it possible for day-to-day life to be entirely serviced by others. The list of staff responsible for the upkeep of George V or George VI was considerable; despite changes in life-styles and expectations among the aristocracy, the numbers of people involved in the presentation of the Queen or Prince Charles still remain considerable. Surrounded by individuals committed to the maintenance of that person, it is little wonder that the individual in question seldom has much sense of the limits between herself or himself and others. The biography of Prince Charles by Jonathan Dimbleby made it clear that working for Prince Charles was no easy matter, since what was expected was total identification and absolute subjection of personal interests together with the maintenance of a critical and competent intelligence.[12] Somewhat unsurprisingly, few people found it possible to enter into this relationship, and, as with the staff of the Princess of Wales and the Duchess of York, the turnover of staff was exceptionally high. Not only, as it appears, are the individuals themselves unstable (or at least erratic), but more importantly, the position which they are being asked to occupy is untenable in the late twentieth century. The general decline in deference, the democratisation of some social attitudes and aspirations, and the determined republicanism of sections of the press all contribute to a situation in which being royal involves compromises, choices and competences impossible to create within a family rooted in hierarchical privilege.

Thus the 'missing persons' of royal biography, and indeed of royalty itself, are the individual kings, queens, princes and princesses socialised into a role and largely out of any meaningful selfhood. In this, they provide an extraordinarily interesting collective example of the possibilities of the distortion and the evasion of human personality. The children brought up by Queen Victoria and George V were all taught to remember, first and foremost, that their parents were royal. The routine curtsies to the parents, the powerful (and in some cases lasting) relationships with nannies, the incarceration in boarding schools and enforced separation from home (or in this case homes) all point to a childhood and adolescence lived in the pursuit of one end, that of maintaining the monarchy. It is this often ruthless determination to preserve the monarchy that is one of the most striking features of the House of Windsor, and paradoxically, that very determination, with the dehumanisation and destabilisation of the individuals concerned, which has done the most to undermine it and to create a monarchy which is now, in many ways, a parody of itself. This pursuit of power has been clearest at times of family crisis and is not merely a feature of recent years. Two examples illustrate the possible ruthlessness of the Windsors: the first was George V's very explicit and determined refusal of help to his cousin Tsar Nicholas II of Russia after the Russian Revolution. Kenneth Rose writes:

> In retrospect, the King's refusal to help his Russian cousins seems wholly out of character; it becomes intelligible only in the context of an England burdened by war-weariness and discontent. The first principle of an hereditary monarchy is to survive; and never was King George V obliged to tread the path of self-preservation more cautiously than in 1917. He felt himself doubly menaced: by a whispering campaign that doubted his patriotism, and by an upsurge of republicanism . . . The King particularly feared the consequences of inviting the Tsar's wife to England, holding her largely responsible for the present state of chaos that exists in Russia.[13]

This legitimation of George V's behaviour makes quite explicit the fragility of the throne. It is apparent from the account in Rose that the government of the day would not have stood in the way of help for the Tsar and his family. Indeed, given the closeness of the family tie, it is quite likely that the help would have been regarded as a perfectly normal form of assistance within the context of family obligations. But George V took an active part in the decision and was clearly the major figure in deciding to leave the Tsar to his fate. After the murder of the Tsar, the King wrote in his diary: 'I hear from Russia that there is every probability that Alicky and four daughters and little boy were murdered at the same time as Nicky. It is too horrible and shows what fiends these Bolshevists are. For poor Alicky, perhaps it was best so. But those poor innocent children.'[14]

The whole affair, of the ruthless prioritisation of King George's interests above those of family was, as Rose points out, a very sensitive matter. It was sensitive not only in the obvious sense of the diplomatic and strategic complications of Britain seeming to aid a deposed and despised ruler and thus affecting in a negative way relations with the new government, but sensitive in the more complex way of exposing the priorities of the monarch. By 1917, George V (and indeed the monarchy in general) was seen by many people to represent, or to aspire to represent, certain consensual national values among which family ties and loyalties would be paramount. Within this set of expectations it would be naturally assumed that the unfortunate in the family should be aided and helped, regardless of other interests. The sensitivity of the court and the government of the day to the whole problem of the Tsar demonstrates the uneasy negotiation which occurred, and the resolution which put the maintenance of the status quo above any humanitarian concerns.

A second example of the Windsors' absolutely ruthless determination to protect the monarchy at all costs can be seen in the marginalisation of Edward VIII and the Duchess of Windsor after the Abdication. The case has an interesting contemporary parallel, in that one of the issues at the forefront of the family dispute was the title 'Her Royal Highness'. In short, Edward VIII assumed that it would be automatically granted to his wife. As the person responsible for deciding who was a Royal Highness and who was not, George VI (and even more so his wife) was determined that the duchess should never be elevated to this status. Family boundaries were to be strictly maintained. So in 1936, just as in 1996, marriage to the wrong person, or divorce, separated an individual forever from the particular status of royalty.

The issue of the title of 'Her Royal Highness' remained alive throughout the lives of the Duke and Duchess of Windsor. Some of the feeling of the Royal Family about the Duchess of Windsor is apparent in the following letter which Queen Mary wrote in 1949:

> I cannot tell you how grieved I am at your brother being so tiresome about the HRH. Giving *her* this title would be fatal, and after all these years I fear lest people think that we condoned this dreadful marriage which has been such a blow to us all in every way. I hope you will be very firm and refuse to do anything about it, and that the Government will back you up. I was grieved that Leopold of the Belgians and his wife saw quite a lot of her in the south of France lately, but she is so pushing and she leaves no stone unturned to remain a thorn in our sides and advertise herself whenever she can. I feel furious that she is over here now, so unnecessary and tactless, and that you should be bothered in this way makes me furious, and I beg and beseech you to be very firm and refuse what he wants . . . with 2 husbands living still, I can't think how D can be so tactless.[15]

But 'D' (Edward VIII) did continue to be tactless, and for the rest of his life he pursued his campaign to try to gain acceptance (both symbolic and real) for his wife.

Yet that acceptance never came, and the title so long aspired to was never allowed. In rather different circumstances, the title of 'Her Royal Highness' was removed from the Princess of Wales in 1996 following her divorce from Prince Charles. The royal club had once again shown that it had very clear expectations about who should, or should not be, a member of the group, and there is no space – either in 1936 or 1996 – for individuals who do not entirely accept the conventional model of behaviour. That model includes, most crucially, a complete separation (in terms of both titles and behaviour) between the royal person and the others. The need for this separation has been recognised quite explicitly from Queen Victoria onwards, and the words 'our position' were seldom absent from her letters. But at the same time as this queen had a strong sense of her position, she also had a strong sense of identity with her subjects, and that sense of identity could be seen in her praise for the modest, the simple and the unpretentious. While far from refusing hierarchy, she also endorsed a suspicion of the uncritical limits of hierarchy, social regulation and exclusion. This aspect of her understanding of the monarchy became most apparent in her correspondence with her eldest daughter, who married into the Prussian Royal Family. To Queen Victoria, this court never failed to offend in its over-rigid protocol, its absurd veneration for birth, and above all its identity with a ruling class. Naturally suspicious of what she regarded as a feckless and dissolute English aristocracy, the queen had little time for a foreign monarchy which actively endorsed a particular social group.[16]

Unfortunately for her descendants, it cannot be said that the British monarchy has continued in Victoria's pattern, and students and biographers of the British monarchy have thus been left with the complex problem of discussing the relationship of the British monarchy to the British class system. Victoria's brilliant negotiation of class relations – by making herself and the monarchy separate from the aristocracy and identifiable with national virtues rather than those derived from class – was overturned by Edward VII and George VI, both of whom located themselves firmly within an aristocratic milieu, with aristocratic associations and, in terms of Edward VII's sexual morality, aristocratic habits. This identification was singularly unfortunate, given the decline in the aristocracy, in terms of both social and material position, from the end of the nineteenth century onwards. As David Cannadine has pointed out, many aspects of aristocratic life were severely curtailed after the First World War: political privilege disappeared, and this was accompanied by shifts within capitalism which made the maintenance of large estates and large households untenable.[17] So the class with which the Royal Family had come to identify themselves disappeared, at least in the socially visible sense. But this left the Royal Family as the representatives of a vanished class, and a vanished life-style. The first crisis provoked by the problems of social identity for the Royal Family was that of Edward VIII's enthusiasm for modernity and the United States. For this Prince of Wales, the appeal of the United States was its greater social informality and 'modern' social habits and behaviour.

The problems of the relationship of the Royal Family to modernity and democracy were solved in the short term by George VI, who chose to identify himself with that most modern of icons, the nuclear family. In the years of the Second World War and the period immediately afterwards this identification was successful. Unfortunately for all concerned, it depended on a patriarchal structure, and the stresses that have been evident in less exalted families when shifts in gendered power relations have taken place have also been apparent in the Royal Family. The evident dedication of the present queen to the role of being royal left little time for motherhood, while the marginality of the position of Prince Philip led to an exaggerated masculinity and evident terror at the idea of female power. Most crucially, in terms of the stability of this particular family, as the country and the culture moved slowly towards more egalitarian family and domestic relations, and a greater emotional literacy (particularly in terms of the recognition of the long-term damage inflicted on children by their separation from their mothers), so the Windsors clung resolutely to the refusal of these changes.

The results are only too apparent in the wreckage of royal marriages and the evident bitterness and misery caused to all concerned by the trials of being royal. Despite optimistic accounts by enthusiasts for the royal family (for example by Frank Prochaska), there is no evidence to suggest that the House of Windsor has been adapting to change or even taking into account the possible changes in personal and family life that have shifted expectations for all their subjects.[18] Faced with this resolute determination to maintain a particular social position in a particular way, royal biographers have chosen two paths: one is to make their subject an exceptional person who somehow enhanced and enriched the position of monarch; the other is to argue that the position of monarch was in some way too great a burden for the individual. The majority of biographies fall into the first group, if only because the majority of British monarchs, from the time of Victoria onwards, did at least fulfil the minimal expectations of the role. As such, the biographies might more appropriately be studies of the role of monarch rather than the person of the monarch, but such is the personalising imperative of biography that it is always the person, rather than the structure and pressures surrounding him or her, who receives attention. On the fringes of accounts of monarchs are the servants and courtiers who made possible the monarch's life; they seldom appear as individuals but as functionaries with specific responsibilities and duties. The immense panoply of monarchy, the machine that makes it feasible for a king or queen, is therefore given little attention; the person of the monarch is of central concern. Where the monarch falls into the category of inadequate, the emphasis on their person is even more exaggerated. Attempting to sum up Edward VIII, Philip Ziegler discusses him thus:

> For those of a certain age Ethelred will always be unready, Edward a Confessor, William a Conqueror, Richard a Lion Heart. How should one describe Edward VIII under such a system? Edward the Unworthy, the unkind might say, yet to do so would beg some fundamental questions, for while it might be argued that he was unworthy of the throne, it has also been maintained that no throne could have been worth the price he was required to pay for it.[19]

This assessment gets close to the emotional reality of the monarchy, the extraordinarily high expectations imposed upon the monarch. In this sense, a rereading of royal biographies might well be in terms of the evidence which they give of their subject's resistance to the demands of monarchy. The 'great' monarch might then well be Queen Victoria or Edward VII, rather than George V or George VI, in that the former pair, rather more than the latter, managed to forge for themselves an identity distinct from their social position. But they did so in times which allowed diverse identities, whereas the twentieth century has been in many ways more rigid in its expectations of the monarch. But the paradox, and indeed in some cases the tragedy of the paradox, is that the creation of a competent and clearly defined individual self demands precisely the kind of care and emotional stability that has seldom been given to the monarchy's children. Stability in the sense of social rigidity and conformity is clearly present, but stability in the sense of close figures with whom to identify is quite another matter. The struggle of the late Princess of Wales to maintain close links with her children, at least by the standard of the Windsors, was symptomatic of a 'modern' attitude to child-rearing which was demonstrably at odds with the expectations of her mother-in-law and to a large extent her husband.

The British created in the Windsors a monarchy which at one time had important unifying advantages. But that ability to be a unifying symbol was one which depended on a deferential social and national culture, and one with certain clear continuities around the issues of family and sexuality. By the end of twentieth century all these certainties have disappeared or become more diverse. In this situation the monarch cannot help but represent partiality and particularity: there is no way in which the monarchy can represent the key characteristics of diversity and difference, since no individual is capable of this multiple representation. Thus the monarchy must be doomed to become a symbol of the past. (The present Queen, despite the best efforts of Ben Pimlott and Sarah Bradford to provide a sympathetic self, personifies precisely that identification. The limited and rigid range of response – starkly visible at the time of the funeral of Princess Diana – graphically illustrated a figure located in a vanished world.) It is thus inevitable that accounts of the monarchy fall into two forms: the deferential and the revelatory, the traditional and the contemporary mode. To write about the monarch in any other way demands a divorce from the twin pillars of conventional biography – the literal chronology and the individualised focus. To allow another form of biography, which fuses the individual and the system, would be transgressive of both the biographical form and the deference still allowed to royalty. Biographies of the royals remain, therefore, locked into the expectations of conventional biography, a double constraint on lives which are already deeply distorted by imposed imperatives.

Chapter 4

Boys' tales

Biographical accounts of the lives of members of the British Royal Family consistently demonstrate the limits of the discussion of gender in conventional biography. That is, that becoming 'male' or 'female', perhaps the most important aspect of identity with which every individual has to deal, is of marginal importance in these accounts. Even when it is apparent, as in the case of Edward VIII, that sexual identity was a highly problematic aspect of the life of this person, the issue is given scant attention. Somehow or other, it is tacitly assumed, the subject became 'a man' and at that point solved, and closed, all discussion of the issue. Obviously, in the case of Edward VIII, the sexual partners in question were a disruptive and unfortunate element in his life, but that they were women is taken for granted. What this suggests is part of the rigid definition often to be found in biography: the individual (unlike any other individual) is not ambiguous and prismatic in his or her relationships with others, but somehow fixed and capable of discovery and revelation. This terror of ambiguity, contradiction and the absence of definition then intrudes into all aspects of the biography; the author is concerned to find the fixed point in any encounter and to see, not the complexity of human relations, but the possible simplicity.

This search for a personal narrative of revelation and clarity has long been part of Western fiction, and is arguably a form of writing which has been dominated by male assumptions and fantasies about 'order' and 'progress'. The great women writers of the nineteenth century all tell 'stories' in the conventional sense of describing the unfolding of events, but the difference between male and female forms of narrative has been suggested by many feminist critics in terms of the relationship of individuals to those events.[1] Thus in narratives by male authors we find women characters who pursue their aims and ambitions regardless of others; indeed the 'others' are protagonists rather than participants in life history. Moll Flanders and Becky Sharpe are typical 'male' heroines; Maggie Tulliver and Fanny Price more typical of the female imagination in their interrelationships with others. Within male narrative fiction we commonly find a less well developed sense of the ties between individuals, and still less the emotional effect of relationships between individuals. The masculine project, certainly in the nineteenth century, was one of the achievement of autonomy and individualism. To be subject to others (the mother and the wife being, of course, the most likely candidates for the entrapment of men) suggested a weakness and vulnerability which was incompatible with conventional masculinity.

This ordering of the ideal of the masculine can be seen in such nineteenth-century agents of male socialisation as the public schools and the armed services. Yet just as these institutions sought to create autonomous, emotionally inexpressive individuals, the inevitable paradox is that they achieved the exact opposite and were the locus of deep, affectionate relationships between men. Many accounts of public schooldays include memories of close, homosexual or quasi-homosexual relationships, which were often abandoned only with difficulty in later life. Clearly, these institutional settings for homosexual relationships, then as now, affected only a small percentage of the relevant age-group, but given the impact which that group had, in terms of cultural and political influence, their experiences are not unimportant. What emerges (and had emerged by the 1920s) was a highly ambivalent attitude to single-sex institutions among the intellectual and cultural elite. The Auden generation, no less than the Bloomsbury group before them, made no secret of their loathing of the public schools and the ethos of upper-class masculinity within which they had been socialised. At the same time, from this single-sex culture had emerged strong, valued friendships between men which were often given priority over relations with women. Thus, although the conditions in which homosexuality was fostered were the subject of criticism, homosexuality itself was regarded with sympathy by a large section of the British cultural elite in the years before the Second World War. Indeed, homosexuality, 'the buggers' as the Bloomsbury group described others and themselves, was in itself an oppositional and transgressive choice – not just in sexual terms, but in terms of the whole climate of conventional masculinity.

In Chapter 3, the rigid masculinity of the British Royal Family (then and now) was seen as a key feature in the inevitable decline and disruptions within that family. For the rest of the country, those neither royal nor subjected to a public school education, masculinity was no less essential to the male person, but less rigidly and formally defined. From the biographies and autobiographies which we have about men in the first forty years of the twentieth century, we can see that the expectations of masculinity were highest among the military and the court and, at another place in the social world, among men in manual occupations which depended upon physical strength and ties to others. In occupations such as mining and fishing, contemporary evidence suggests that the sexes lived in different worlds, and that those worlds had very clear labels of masculine and feminine. When D.H. Lawrence wrote his thinly disguised autobiography in *Sons and Lovers*, he described that separation, not just of function but also of subjectivity and emotional experience, between the lives of women and men.[2] The idea of the companionate marriage, which historians and sociologists have seen as a key feature of Western societies in the twentieth century, was hardly present in Lawrence, or in those families whose reality was reflected in his novel.

The question raised by Lawrence, and raised by him in terms

which directly challenged the tolerance of homosexuality among the Bloomsbury group, was the ancient question of the terms of relations between the sexes put into the context of the evident empowerment of women at the end of the nineteenth century and the fracturing of the Victorian ideal of dependent femininity. Like many others, Lawrence recognised that this ideal was as much a fantasy as a reality; but the question still remained for him, as it did for other men, of how to accept the strength of women without perceiving that strength as a threat to a carefully (and probably tenuously) achieved masculinity. Around this issue, and the issue of attitudes to homosexuality, can be observed one of the crucial divisions of autobiography and biography about, and by, men in the twentieth century. One tradition, in the twentieth century as much as the nineteenth century, was that of the complete refusal of anything problematic about the resolution of sexual identity. Then and now, men (and to a lesser extent women) have proved capable of writing their autobiographies – and biographies of other men – as if this crucial element and stage in human development and aspect of human existence needed no comment. Shelves of this material exist. But in other traditions – more notably in autobiography and in that fiction which is close to autobiography – men have openly described their homosexual relationships, and made no secret of the complexity of their sexual lives. In particular, what becomes clear in reading some fiction is that homosexuality is in some sense a necessary step to emotional understanding and maturity. The denial of this feeling, and the refusal of the recognition of the strength of ties between men, carries with it a refusal of emotional life which is deeply destructive of creativity.

These tensions around sexuality, and around the expressive and the inexpressive, run with a clear and definable presence throughout twentieth-century auto/biography by, and about, men. Indeed, it would be no exaggeration to say that, because there is a greater suspicion of affectivity and emotional expression among men (whether homosexual or not), male auto/biography is dominated by a denial of emotional and sexual life.

'Keeping the feminine at bay' could be the banner under which a number of the great male writers of the twentieth century worked. (Nor were writers in any sense an exceptional group; men as politicians, journalists and soldiers all exhibit the same degree of distance, often fearful distance, from women.) In the case of one of the writers discussed here, George Orwell, his evident homophobia (accompanied by an equal wariness of women) will be suggested as a determining element in Orwell's social and political analysis.

Of all British writers in the twentieth century, Orwell has achieved the greatest integration into the general culture. *Animal Farm* and *Nineteen Eighty-Four* are widely regarded as classics, and often read and described as factual accounts of the future. The terms 'Orwellian' and 'Big Brother' are widely used to describe the particular forms of centralised state politics which were Orwell's targets. The reasons for the integration, and indeed the appropriation, of Orwell by Western culture are thus not difficult to identify: his work fits into the post-1945 politics of the West and the general condemnation, in Western politics, of state socialism and most particularly of state socialism as practised in the Soviet Union. Many people have pointed out that Orwell had no intention of attacking socialism *per se* in his work. His intention was certainly to condemn certain forms of political authoritarianism, but the identification of this form of politics with socialism was not his. Orwell lived and died a socialist, the argument continues, but one who had conducted a life-long feud with the Communist parties of both Britain and the Soviet Union. His political opinions were summed up in his own words as 'democratic socialism', and his social vision was one in which the ideas of 'decency' and 'the ordinary' were paramount.[3]

Yet these words carry with them numerous coded messages, and in order to interpret Orwell we have to recognise that what lay at the centre of his social vision was an essentially heterosexual, and conventional, social model in which women were both unproblematic, in that they were assumed to be just like men, and deeply problematic, in the sense that at any moment they might become a definably different sex. The women in the early fiction (*A Clergyman's Daughter* and *Keep the Aspidistra Flying*) are either put upon by men, or put upon them.[4] Exploited or harridan, women never appear as capable of any agency other than that related to either the acceptance or denial of male choices. In Orwell's autobiographical writing – *Homage to Catalonia, Down and Out in Paris and London* and *The Road to Wigan Pier* – there are almost no women. The few exceptions are the unnamed mother in the contented domestic interior in *The Road to Wigan Pier* and the overworked cook in *Down and Out in Paris and London.* Thus:

> In a working-class home – I am not thinking at the moment of the unemployed, but of comparatively prosperous homes – you breathe a warm, decent, deeply human atmosphere which is not so easy to find elsewhere . . . Especially on winter evenings after tea, when the fire glows in the open range and dances mirrored in the steel fender, when Father, in shirt-sleeves, sits in the rocking chair at one side of the fire reading the racing finals, and Mother sits on the other with sewing . . . it is a good place to be in . . .[5]

and the second woman, hard at work in a Parisian restaurant:

> The cook and I generally found time to eat our dinner between ten and eleven o'clock. At midnight the cook would steal a packet of food for her husband, stow it under her clothes, and make off, whimpering that these hours would kill her and she would give notice in the morning.[6]

These women we have to note, have obviously worked hard and long, and yet their reward, in Orwell's view, is a place as a stage character in the working-class home or as a 'whimpering' cook in the Paris kitchen. That 'whimpering' cook, we must remember, has just worked an eighteen hour day, in conditions which Orwell describes as those of slavery.

The inference that can be drawn from the portrayals of these women is that Orwell had no false chivalry in his relations with women: they could work as hard as men, and there is no outrage in Orwell's description of the amount of work demanded of the Parisian cook. In much the same way, Orwell made few allowances for his wife in terms of either her work or her emotional life. When Eileen Orwell's much-loved brother was killed at Dunkirk, Orwell showed no outward sign of anything approaching sympathy or understanding. Even a sympathetic biographer of Orwell was forced to write defensively of this attitude:

> There is little in Orwell's letters or diaries that would indicate that his wife was in such pain. He did not talk about such things to other people, and he would not have agonised over it even in his private diaries. There can be no question that he felt her pain and was moved by it, but he took a stoical attitude toward such things and was not prepared to deal with them in the open. He was always so careful to keep his emotions under control, at least on the outside, but no one can read very far in his works without realising that the passive expression he was inclined to present to the outside world marked deeply felt passions. *So much of his upbringing* had encouraged him to guard his feelings, to keep his thoughts to himself. This conditioning may have sharpened his powers of observation, but it did little to help him deal openly with emotional difficulties of the kind that Eileen's situation presented after her brother's death.[7]

The italics here are mine, and are given to emphasise that although Orwell *became* exceptional, and is known as one of the great Western writers of the twentieth century, the circumstances and conditions which shaped him, and which moulded his attitude to emotional life, were ordinary ones. The circumstances were not literally commonplace – no education which included Eton could be described as that – but they were circumstances shared by a generation of middle- and upper middle-class British males. Within this experience there was a general prohibition on emotional expressivity and a homophobia in part produced by the segregation of the sexes. In this sense, therefore, Orwell's upbringing was 'ordinary' and was one he shared with hundreds of other people of his class, race and gender.

But so powerful was the force of this socialisation that both biographers and writers of autobiography have often failed to observe its results or to emphasise the degree to which a rigid separation was constructed between the public and private worlds of individuals. Orwell, Waugh and, in a later generation, Philip Larkin were all men whose initial social experience of the world was provided by all-male institutions. Orwell and Waugh received the traditional boarding school educations of men of their class, and one of Orwell's most famous essays remains 'Such, Such were the Joys', his account of his preparatory school.[8] The figure who can still strike horror into the reader is that of the headmaster's wife, the redoubtable Mrs Wilkes, who quite appropriately 'traced her family's origins back to some fierce clan in Scotland' and according to Orwell was a monster of cruelty and sadism. The point is not whether this was true, but the absence in Orwell and his biographers of any comment which might suggest that, to an eight-year-old boy, any woman who was not his mother, and yet appeared to act as one, would be the object of suspicion, fear and rage. However sympathetic to Orwell's plight at prep school his biographers are (and both Bernard Crick and Michael Shelden allow that Orwell was unhappy there), there nevertheless remains an attitude which is characteristic of the culture of masculinity, in that it was Orwell's response to the prep school, rather that the prep school itself, which was problematical. Thus, for example, Shelden quotes Mrs Wilkes's own view of Orwell that 'There was no warmth in him', and both Shelden and Crick cite Cyril Connolly's memories of the same school as perfectly happy, or at least acceptable ones.[9] What is being achieved here is a normalisation of a particular kind of masculine socialisation, a normalisation which had such obvious results in Orwell's relationship with women and limited emotional response that it would seem worth comment.

But in general men writing about men, and men writing about themselves, do not investigate the nature of the origin of their relationships with others. That project of masculinity, which emphasises autonomy and the completed self, does not fit easily with subjective or reflective accounts of the origin of the person, or even the unknowability of the person. Given that men such as Larkin, Orwell and Waugh were all fundamentally concerned with establishing particular voices that could be immediately identified as their own, there is little encouragement or even perceived need to review the way in which that public voice is being constructed in order to mask or to express, or to be a substitute for, more immediate emotional expressivity. Psycho-analysis has long recognised the ways in which individuals attempt to make good psychic damage through creative work: it is a theory which fits closely the events of the lives of many major male writers.[10] What is even more striking about these individuals is their refusal of the acknowledgement of subjective expression in the construction and genesis of their work. Unlike women, who are generally more likely to account for creativity in ways related to their emotional and personal experiences, men will frequently refuse this association.

Orwell wrote little in his later life that was as autobiographical as *The Road to Wigan Pier*, *Down and Out in Paris and London* and *Homage to Catalonia*. In his essays published during the Second World War, he emphasised his enthusiasm for England, and for its domestic fabric. At the same time he repeatedly condemned that particular kind of socialist whom he clearly associated (like D.H. Lawrence) with the Bloomsbury group. Homophobia was alive and well in Orwell in later life, just as much as it was in his youth. Yet at the same time, his writing expresses little enthusiasm for literal femininity – there is almost nothing in either his fiction or his non-fiction that explicitly praises women, their appearance or the possibilities of the feminine as distinct from the masculine. As it is, what we have in Orwell is a view of the

world, and an account of it, which virtually excludes the feminine. The artefacts of English life which Orwell constantly
praises are those of masculine experience. Equally, his account of
'abroad' is largely in terms of its discomfort. In ways which are
very similar to Larkin, Orwell had almost no sympathy for countries other than England. Orwell was prepared to fight for
Republican Spain, but *Homage to Catalonia* gives little account of
the subjective experience of Spain. Nor does it evoke anything
like the response we can find in Gerald Brenan, whose writing at
about the same time as Orwell expressed a greater and deeper
knowledge of Spanish culture.[11]

Yet if we substitute 'subjectivity' for 'culture' here, we can perhaps begin to see ways in which Orwell's view of the world –
identified so firmly as it is with the material and the literal – is so
typical of the kind of understanding deemed appropriate for
masculinity. Brenan, with his bisexuality and his relationship to
the Bloomsbury group, represents a definably different tradition,
and to a certain extent a much more radical one than Orwell in
that he is prepared to see the possibilities of understandings of
the world that are different from his own. In his sympathy with
non-Protestant, and indeed non-Anglo-Saxon cultures, Brenan is
much closer to Evelyn Waugh, whose writing about 'abroad'
often reaches heights of inspired lyricism, while Orwell's descriptions of non-English countries emphasise the dirt, the poverty
and the disease. In seeing these things, and in refusing the roman-
ticism of some accounts of Europe, Orwell provides a salutary
correction to rose-coloured accounts of European and other
civilisations. But again, we can see a pattern emerging in the
masculine relationship to the world outside the British Isles: on
the one side are writers such as E.M. Forster, Waugh and Brenan,
who find in Europe (and beyond) a sensuality which they cannot
locate in England. For Orwell and Larkin, masculinity begins
and ends in England; not untypically both were drawn, in their
later years, to bleak and deserted landscapes.

These personal agendas, involving both literally and symbolically 'placing' their masculinity, can be seen to dominate the lives of all the writers named above. The crucial distinction between the writers can be identified as their toleration of their own, or those of others, relations with people of their own sex. Waugh, in *A Little Learning*, made little secret of his adolescent love for other boys, and was prepared to admit in his diaries and letters that he enjoyed the company of men.[12] At the same time (and despite ritual comments about certain kinds of blatant homosexuality), he is tolerant about different kinds of masculinity. Indeed, his deepest fictional contempt is reserved for his most conventionally masculine characters, such as Rex Mottram in *Brideshead Revisited*. In his description of Rex Mottram, Waugh expresses both his dislike of what he sees as modern manners (particularly when North American in origin) with the kind of ruthless desire for order and 'improvement' which he sees Mottram as personifying. What is particularly interesting about the forms of masculinity set out for the reader in *Brideshead Revisited* is that, although Waugh makes his hero Charles Ryder an artist and an 'expressive' man, he also assigns to him a rejection of certain forms of artistic choice. It is part of Ryder's movement towards maturity, therefore, that he explicitly abandons the symbols of allegiance to the Bloomsbury group. In his youth, Ryder buys without any self-consciousness works by Bloomsbury artists:

> On my first afternoon I proudly hung a reproduction of Van Gogh's *Sunflowers* over the fire and set up a screen, painted by Roger Fry with a Provençal landscape, which I had bought inexpensively when the Omega workshops were sold up . . . My books were meagre and commonplace – Roger Fry's *Vision and Design*, the Medici Press edition of *A Shropshire Lad*, *Eminent Victorians* . . .[13]

But as he acquires new friends, and new tastes, a different perception emerges:

> I had nursed a love of architecture, but, though in opinion I

had made that easy leap, characteristic of my generation, from the puritanism of Ruskin to the puritanism of Roger Fry, my sentiments at heart were insular and medieval.

This was my conversion to the baroque. Here under that high and insolent dome, under those coffered ceilings; here, as I passed through those arches and broken pediments to the pillared shade beyond and sat, hour by hour, before the fountain, probing its shadows, tracing its lingering echoes, rejoicing in all its clustered feats of daring and invention, I felt a whole new system of nerves alive within me, as though the water that spurted and bubbled among its stones, was indeed a life-giving spring.[14]

It is equipped with this new understanding that Ryder can meet, and assess, Rex Mottram in terms other than those of straight-forward admiration for his success in the masculine world of high finance and politics. In a scene in a Parisian restaurant Waugh sets out a brilliant duet between Ryder and Mottram in which two attitudes to the world are played out over the successive courses of French bourgeois cooking. Rex Mottram's view of the food is analogous to his attitude to the world: endless interference and inability to recognise that simplicity and excellence are often possible. Thus:

The sole was so simple and unobtrusive that Rex failed to notice it . . . I closed my mind to him as best I could and gave myself to the food before me, but sentences came breaking in on my happiness, recalling me to the harsh, acquisitive world which Rex inhabited.[15]

Charles Ryder and Rex Mottram share that meal just before Mottram marries Julia, the woman whom Ryder is subsequently to love. As Ryder notes on that evening, Mottram's attitude to Julia is that of purchase ('He wanted a woman: he wanted the best on the market . . .'), and it is this attitude, of the incursion of commercial and monetary values into human relationships, that provides the focus for Waugh's conservative (but not Conserva-tive) critique of modern society. *Brideshead Revisited* is fiction, and thus must fall outside the subject of auto/biography, but it is essential reading for any understanding of Waugh and his poli-tics, since it provides such a powerful credo for his readers. In particular, what it does is to suggest an account of the possibilities of intervention in the social world which calls into question many of the taken-for-granted assumptions of the later part of the twentieth century. Central to these assumptions was the idea, dating from the Enlightenment, that society could be ordered and arranged by human effort and considered judgement. The acceptance of planning and of constructing the social order were both crucial ingredients in the complex of ideas that has been described as modernity and the post-Enlightenment para-digm. Indeed, the nineteenth-century project of masculinity was directly and intimately associated with these ideas, in that 'masculine' science, reason and technology were pivotal ele-ments in the idea of controlling and harnessing the natural world.

But as the twentieth century proceeded, and certainly as a result of the First World War and even more fundamentally the Second, visible cracks began to appear in this identification of masculinity with the ideals of social progress and social order. The First World War made it plain that conventional masculinity could result, not in progress but in disaster, and that the refusal of this conventional model was more rational than blind obedience. The Second World War made the possibilities of planning and social order even more problematic; as numerous critiques have argued, one result of the Enlightenment was Auschwitz.[16] Every person in every society in the West has been affected by that historical progression, but for men, more so than women, the progression has posed complex and so far insolvable problems about the nature of identification with historical and social change and the very nature of reason. Precisely because men made the project of the Enlightenment so singularly their own, the difficulties of resolving that relationship are to be found most clearly in men's auto/biographical writing. For women there remains the issue of finding a personal voice that can transcend the limits of the private space, but there is no intricate relationship to the dominant discourses of the public world to be unravelled, if only because women have largely not participated so fully in that public space.

Thus we can see Waugh's resistance to modernity as part of a central theme and dilemma of the twentieth century: of how men, and masculinity, can relocate themselves in relationship to a God of Reason (and/or Rationality) who has so demonstrably produced human misery. Waugh's solution was a recourse to Roman Catholicism and with it a culture of experience and understanding which seemed to offer resources not available in the secular world. As a later Roman Catholic novelist, David Lodge, was to remark of a fictional character who was converted to Catholicism: 'Catholicism, to which Michael introduced her, seemed to be just what she was looking for: it was subtle, it was urbane, it had history, learning, art (especially music) on its side.'[17] Much the same could be said of Waugh's understanding of Catholicism: it offered an alternative both to Reason (and with it resistance to those projects of social transformation and social order to which Waugh was instinctively as well as politically unsympathetic) and to the values and standards of what he perceived as the dominant traditions within English culture. Rex Mottram represents all the more unacceptable aspects of the twentieth-century world: his values are dominated by the capitalist market-place, and his attitudes to individuals and experiences are ruthlessly exploitative.

Thus to read *Brideshead Revisited* simply as reactionary overlooks the novel's position within a set of debates and discussions which are pivotal to the twentieth century, and to the place of men and masculinity within it. *Brideshead Revisited* is set at the end of the Second World War, and an aspect of that war which is crucial to the understanding of gender relations in the twentieth century is the way in which it served to preserve and rescue a certain version of masculinity – that associated with physical courage and

military valour.[18] To fight for one's country had become, after the
First World War, a contested position. That war had been contentious from the start and by its conclusion had revealed the
colossal shortcomings of the conventional model of military
masculinity. The growth of vocal pacifism in the 1920s and the
explicit dissent by a generation of men from the idea of fighting
for their country had made anti-militarism very much an
accepted position in the inter-war years. Orwell, like others of his
generation, had fought for the Republicans in Spain, but this
commitment was about a specific political allegiance rather than
a taken-for-granted acceptance of militarism. The fight against
fascism of 1939–45, therefore, in part reinvented the idea of a
credible military: despite considerable argument about how the
war should be conducted, there was little dissent from the idea
that the war was inherently just and worth fighting.

Little wonder, then, that masculinity emerged from the battle-
grounds of Europe in 1945 with a model that would once again
include physical strength and an ideal of heroism. This revival
played, in the 1950s, a considerable part in the idealogical
reconstruction of gender relations, which were to become both
traditional and conservative. The shifts towards a greater social
equality between the sexes were slowed, as both Britain and the
United States endorsed models of nuclear families in which
female economic dependence on men was taken for granted and
women's integration into the public world slowed down. One of
the fiercest quasi-autobiographical attacks of these expectations
of gender relations came in Sylvia Plath's *The Bell Jar*.[19] Writing
of a childhood and adolescence in the white suburbs of the
United States she wrote:

> When I was nineteen, pureness was the great issue. Instead
> of the world being divided up into Catholics and Protestants
> or Republicans and Democrats or white men and black
> men or even men and women, I saw the world divided into
> people who had slept with somebody and people who
> hadn't.[20]

A view elaborated and endorsed by the lampooned character Buddy Willard:

> He was always saying how his mother said, 'What a man wants is a mate and what a woman wants is infinite security,' and 'what a man is is an arrow into the future and what a woman is is the place the arrow shoots off from.'[21]

In an important sense *The Bell Jar* is a devastating attack on the values of the post-war Western world, and in particular those of the suburban United States. Plath's whole life could be read as an attempt to challenge (as her contemporary and compatriot Anne Sexton did) the consequences for women of the kind of society aspired to by the Buddy Willards of her world, a society that had a rigid gender hierarchy and refused complications of sexual ambiguity in the same way that it refused political dissent and social deviance.[22] But what Plath and Sexton both did in their generation was to show the possibility of female refusal of this culture; without any explicit political statement in their work they challenged the assumption that male authority and male presence was in any sense definitive and authoritative.[23] In doing this, they contributed (although only indirectly) to the wave of women's writing that was to emerge in the late 1960s and early 1970s and become known collectively as 'second-wave feminism'. Yet just as this tradition was being forged (it can be illustrated in the works of many authors less well known than either Plath and Sexton), for men the nature of masculinity remained problematic. Endorsing the post-1945 consensus of the masculine meant, to a large extent, endorsing precisely that version of masculinity which excluded women and regained that aspiration of separation and autonomy that had been typical of nineteenth-century masculinity. In Britain (although less so in the United States) identification with militarisation and military aggression was acceptable in wartime but became very much less acceptable in the years after the war, when the class relations of military service became once again less explicitly committed to the preservation of democracy and more explicitly committed to British imperial interests. The Colonel Blimp who had been a joke in the Second World War was rather less so when located in terms of British engagement in Cyprus or Suez.

Precisely because women were so explicitly excluded from the exercise of political power, the public presentation of femininity was less problematic. The media does not (indeed it seldom has, except in the case of mothering) devote attention to the 'crisis' in the behaviour of young women as it repeatedly has in the case of young men. Yet from 1945 onwards, considerable attention has been devoted to the question of 'preserving' masculinity. In Britain in the 1950s, this took the form of debates about the impact of the ending of National Service on young men, and in the 1960s there were discussions throughout the West on the appearance and behaviour of young men who appeared to be challenging every known expectation of masculinity. Long hair, unisex clothing and, in the United States, refusal of military service for the war in Vietnam were all attributed to a decadence within men and masculinity. Much of the debate and public comment was a coded fear about homosexuality: 'going soft' was a frequently cited phrase about the rejection of a particular form of machismo. Feminism made it rapidly clear that, as far as women were concerned, little had actually changed in the behaviour of men. The permissive society, feminist critics argued, was nothing other than a celebration of male-defined heterosexuality.[24]

Within this changing climate about sexuality and gender relations which dates from the early 1960s, auto/biography took an increasingly gendered form. On the one hand, more women were writing auto/biography than ever before, and doing so as part of a culture which explicitly encouraged the emergence of women's voices. On the other, men continued to write the kind of public, deeply conventional auto/biography, that had always been an aspect of male writing. In a very obvious sense, therefore (notwithstanding certain exceptions), women's auto/biographical writing became both more innovative and more radical, while men's remained locked into a rigid distinction

between the public and the private which reflected the problematic nature of late twentieth-century masculinity. As Maya
Angelou and others published their autobiographies, and in
doing so extended the boundaries of the genre, male auto/
biography saw no such corresponding development.[25] It was not
so much that a mass of material, and increasingly revelatory
material, was not published, but rather that the form and the
determining parameters of the material remained largely the
same. Nevertheless, what did begin to emerge in the 1990s were
accounts by men which identified their vulnerability and/or their
sense of marginality from the dominant culture. Hardly surprisingly, much of this writing came from gay men, who had always
had to live a shadowy existence and had had to wait for most
of the twentieth century in order to explore the possibilities of
literary freedom.

The changes in sexual mores and sexual behaviour that
became part of the common culture of the West (and the
changes were emphatically Western rather than global) made it
possible for gay men to discuss openly the nature of their sexuality and its implications in terms of their relations to others. As
Jeffrey Weeks and others have pointed out, there has always been
a substantial literature about the nature of gay relationships and
gay sub-cultures, but until recently it has had to exist in a coded
or submerged form.[26] Little explicit discussion of homosexuality
was possible, even though Western literature is replete with examples of close relationships between men. But the transformations
of the 1960s and 1970s made a new openness and revelation
possible. This was further developed by the identification of the
HIV virus in the 1980s; HIV (and Aids) brought a new, tragic
dimension to autobiography in that many of the men who now
came to write it were themselves either infected or closely
involved with the afflicted.[27]

Yet for all the passion and the emotional intensity which the
auto/biography of Aids brought to the genre, it did not itself
offer transformatory possibilities. Literature by or about the mor-
tally threatened is in itself no new departure within auto/

biography. What is striking, however, about the literature by gay men is that it in many ways conforms to the pattern of previous auto/biography. Clearly, the sexual revelation and the acceptance of the sexually explicit is greater, but what is reserved is the sense of agency and the desire for individual strength and autonomy. The extent to which men will go to maintain what they see as an acceptable exterior self has been widely explored by male writers. Edmund White and Geoffrey Wolff are examples of this genre and as such represent compelling evidence of men's need to maintain a presence acceptable by other men.[28]

But in our reading of the relationship of the real Sylvia Plath (and the fictional Esther Greenwood) to Buddy Willard we are doomed to know that, while Sylvia Plath rejected one unsatisfactory version of masculinity in Buddy, the model of masculinity to which she aspired was no less problematic. Buddy Willard represented what is sometimes known as the 'provider' model of masculinity – a man who regarded the material support of his family as his responsibility and assumed that with this responsibility went a natural authority over its members. For Sylvia Plath's mother, doomed to life-long poorly-paid jobs precisely because of her husband's incompetence at provision, such a man must have seemed an ideal of security and responsibility. But Sylvia and Esther, unlike their real and fictional mothers, could not overlook Buddy's stupidity, his sexual double standards and his overwhelming literal-mindedness. In Buddy Willard there remains forever a picture of the failure of the American imagination, a failure which Henry James had identified at the beginning of the twentieth century but was no less real fifty years later. The particularity of that failure of imagination, in this context, lies less in Buddy's inability to perceive the possibilities of other understandings of the world (although he is markedly deficient in that understanding) than in his rigid and fixed masculinity. The strengths of that version of masculinity (of domestic provision and possible heroism in wartime) mean nothing to Sylvia/Esther. What they pursue is a sense of possibility, of the male heterosexual who unites feminine understanding with male strength.

That vision, and that ideal, arguably dominates relations between women and men throughout the twentieth century. The version of masculinity constructed by white, middle-class Edwardian Britain, the empire-builders model of much school-boy fiction, was largely challenged by the tragedies and the losses of the First World War. But what took its place was often barely different: Virginia Woolf's searing critique of masculinity, *Three Guineas*, was written, we have to remember, not in 1916 but in 1938. By that period in English history she was able to construct the critique, but she could hardly point to any evidence suggesting that the patriarchy that she was attacking had disappeared or was even beginning to disappear. Indeed, in the midst of her family Virginia Woolf lived through continuing evidence of the vitality of patriarchy and its social forms. The case in question was that of the concealed paternity of her niece Angelica Garnett. Angelica's biological father was Duncan Grant, the lover of Virginia Woolf's sister Vanessa Bell. But at the time of Angelica's birth it was thought essential by Vanessa Bell, Duncan Grant and other close friends to conceal Angelica's actual paternity and present her as the child of Vanessa's husband, Clive Bell.[29] This deception (of Angelica, Clive's parents and the world in general) continued until 1937, when Angelica was nineteen. Writing in 1984, Angelica Garnett said of this decision:

> Presumably it was with his approval that Vanessa and Clive decided to ignore the fact that Duncan was my father. It was arranged between them that Duncan, on my arrival in this world, was to telegraph Clive's parents, Mr and Mrs Bell, in Clive's name ... Clive and Vanessa must have made the decision together in a spirit that, lightheartedly, they imagined unconventional – for that is the way it was later presented to me. But parents and parents-in-law have always been misled about such things: given the freedom that Bloomsbury supposed it had won for itself, it is, on the

> contrary, the conventionality of the deception that is
> surprising.[30]

It is indeed, the 'conventionality of the deception' that startles the reader. Yet the very nature of the deception, the question of the identity of the child's father, is one that has been a common theme of English and other literatures for centuries. Mis-taken, mis-understood and mis-placed paternity have provided part of the plot for novelists and dramatists from Shakespeare onwards. A common result of the confusion over paternity is that individuals veer dangerously close to incest. Angelica Garnett did not, in the technical sense, become involved in an incestuous union, but she did marry David Garnett, an ex-lover of her father's.

The web of friendship surrounding David Garnett, Duncan Grant and Vanessa Bell has now been extensively documented. In that it is a part of the history of the Bloomsbury group, it is also a part of English cultural history. Equally, it is a part of that cultural history which involved the emergence of modernism in English literature and the expression of that development in its great voice, Virginia Woolf. But what Virginia Woolf recognised was that the nature of modernism was feminine – not, as she knew, in any literal sense, but in the way in which the condition and experience of twentieth-century urban life offered a range of possibilities, a diversity and in a sense an inherent instability of identity which was closer to the range of possible female experience than the fixed and proscribed nature of masculinity. Woolf's life-long protest against the fixed nature of Edwardian masculinity (a protest which reached its highest point in *Three Guineas*) was to place her forever in the same literary company as Joyce and E.M. Forster and away from the fixed 'masculine' certainties of writers of her generation such as Orwell. Woolf is separated from both Orwell and Waugh by her death before the end of the Second World War: for Orwell and Waugh the experience of surviving the war, and the revelations of the Holocaust and the Stalinist purges, were to make their existing certainties firmer and more resolute.

For neither of these men did their personal circumstances give any doubt about their paternity. Unlike Angelica Garnett, both grew up in homes which were organised around Edwardian values of particular kinds of precision and decorum. In both homes, as their biographers have subsequently revealed, their mothers had a love and concern for the arts and represented a sense of feminine difference which established in their sons a clear, obvious sense of the lines of sexual demarcation. For them, the transition to adult masculinity could be achieved within a completely conventional pattern of masculine and feminine behaviour. But for men growing up in other circumstances, and growing up not with successful masculinity but with problematic masculinity, the personal results were very different, as were the relationships of those individuals to twentieth-century history. Waugh and Orwell, for all their very different ideas about social change and transformation in the twentieth century, nevertheless fundamentally engaged with these phenomena and never turned their backs on the possibilities and implications of global cultures, and in particular the cultural domination of the United States. Two male writers who contrast with this pattern, and who belong to a later generation than Waugh and Orwell, are Philip Larkin and John Osborne. Both these men came from less prosperous and less socially secure backgrounds that Orwell and Waugh, both wrote of difficult relations with women (in both cases their mothers), and both left work – poetry in the case of Larkin and drama in the case of Osborne – which is forever identified with discontent, in particular discontent with the nature and experience of modernity.

In Osborne's two volumes of autobiography, *A Better Class of Person* and *Almost a Gentlemen*, the towering figure on to whom Osborne projects his dissatisfactions is that of his mother.[31] In one of the early descriptions of her in *A Better Class of Person*, Osborne demonstrates in every adjective, the depths of irritation and dislike that his mother aroused in him:

My mother's hair was very dark, occasionally hennaed. Her

face was a floury dark mask, her eyes were an irritable brown, her ears small, so unlike her father's ('He's got Satan's ears, he has'), her nose surprisingly fine. Her remaining front teeth were large, yellow and strong. Her lips were a scarlet-black sliver covered in some sticky shine name Yahiti or Tattoo, which she brought with all her other make-up from Woolworth's.[32]

As the narrative of *A Better Class of Person* proceeds it becomes transparently plain that Nellie Beatrice – as he describes his mother – is ever-present in Osborne's thoughts. In *A Sense of Detachment*, which was first performed in 1972, one of the characters was to say:

Woman is Dead! Long love Woman! I do not believe it. She has always triumphed in my small corner of spirit, just as I have failed her image – my broken, misty, self-deceiving image you may say – during most of my life. And, remembering it, what a long time it has been. I believe in Woman, whatever that may be, just as I believe in God, because they were both invented by man. If I am their inventor, they are my creators, and they will continue to exist.[33]

The depths of Osborne's involvement with women is apparent in both his fiction and his autobiography. He cannot turn his back on Nellie Beatrice, and even when a successful adult he is haunted by the tone of her voice, and as he sees it, the depths of her ignorance and misunderstanding. The deep need and deep fear of Nellie Beatrice, which conforms so clearly to everything Melanie Klein ever said about a child's perception of good and bad mothers, is then projected on to Osborne's wives and women friends.[34] He passionately desires them all, sees in each person the possibility of psychic freedom, and then in each case finds nothing except characteristics to criticise and condemn. The second volume of Osborne's autobiography, an autobiography which had opened with repetitious attacks on the appearance and the understanding of his mother, concludes with pages that attack two of the women once married to Osborne: Jill Bennett and Penelope Gilliatt. Of Jill Bennett, who committed suicide after their marriage ended, Osborne wrote:

> She had no love in her heart for people and only a little more for dogs. Her brand of malignity, unlike Penelope's, went beyond even the banality of ambition. It had its roots deep in a kind of bourgeois criminality. Her frigidity was almost total. She loathed men and pretended to love women, whom she hated even more. She was at ease only in the company of homosexuals, who she also despised but whose narcissism matched her own. I never heard her say an admiring thing of anyone. Her contempt was so petty and terrible. Everything about her life had been a pernicious confection, a sham.[35]

The extent of this misogyny is apparent throughout Osborne's work, even if the obituary for Jill Bennett is the most vituperative attack on one individual. But literary misogyny is, as numerous feminist critics from de Beauvoir to Kate Millett have pointed out, no new thing. Indeed, when Jane Austen wrote in *Persuasion* that the pen has generally been in the hands of men, she was making a similar point about the domination of literature by men and male values.[36] But – and it is an emphatic but – Austen and even de Beauvoir were writing at times when the impact (not to mention the very possibility) of literary modernism was hardly apparent on their respective genres. Austen was writing in a narrative tradition that was profoundly related to the belief in the emancipatory possibility of reason. One hundred and fifty years later de Beauvoir was still fundamentally part of this tradition and this sense of possibility, and there was, in the tradition, an expectation of universal understanding. What this tradition gave to men who occupied positions within its central understanding was prestige and, more importantly, the assurance of representing universal reality. That belief, the very security and assurance of universality, was shattered by literary modernism and by the changes bought about in literature by Joyce and Woolf. These writers shifted the nature of the authorial voice, and with it much else about the relationship of fiction (be it prose or drama) to gender. A significant aspect of literary masculinity became, in the twentieth century, insecure.

Thus for Osborne, as for Larkin and Orwell, women in the general sense became both objects of cruel abuse and the 'signifiers' of much that is socially and culturally problematic. We have already seen that Orwell was deeply hostile to the Bloomsbury group; his comments on the 'sandal wearing' bohemians of his generation are widely quoted. Further, his discussion of mining and the conditions in which miners lived is accompanied by a remark which puts the relationship of the Bloomsbury group to the exploitation of labour in stark terms:

> You and I and the editor of the *Times Lit Supp.*, and the Nancy poets and the Archbishop of Canterbury and Comrade X, author of *Marxism for Infants* – all of us really owe the comparative decency of our lives to poor drudges underground, blackened to the eyes, with their throats full of dust, driving their shovels forward with arms and belly muscles of steel.[37]

Orwell may or may not have known that the financial support for the ménage at Charleston, presided over by Vanessa Bell, came from the inherited wealth of Clive Bell, wealth which was in part derived from mining. Orwell, like Waugh, was very conscious of the need to earn money; despite their backgrounds and public school education, neither of them could depend on unearned income. Throughout the majority of his life, Orwell had little money; Waugh was more financially successful, even if his own habits never guaranteed financial security. But what he was acutely conscious of was his ability to *earn* money. Writing to his future wife, Laura Herbert he said:

> I am restless and moody and misanthropic and lazy and

have no money except what I can earn and if I got ill I would starve. In fact it is a sorry proposition. On the other hand I think I could . . . reform and become quite strict about not getting drunk and I am pretty sure I should be faithful. Also there is always a fair chance that there will be another bigger economic crash in which case if you had married a noble-man with a great house you might find yourself starving, while I am very clever and could probably earn a living of some sort somewhere.[38]

In this assessment Waugh was entirely correct: he was able to support a large family in considerable style (if not luxury) through the power of his pen, while his brother-in-law, Auberon Herbert, the inheritor of considerable wealth, was rendered penniless by a hopeless incompetence with money and the social world.

Thus both Orwell and Waugh made, in the full sense of 'liter-ally', their money and in doing so achieved the competence expected of men and masculinity. So did Osborne and Larkin, but what is different about these two later writers is that they regarded money and the making of it in more problematic ways. Neither Larkin nor Osborne were born to money or had any social experience of inherited wealth; from his earliest writing it is apparent that Larkin is concerned, if not obsessed, with money and financial relationships between individuals. Osborne is simi-larly preoccupied; money as a means of exchange and indeed of understanding is ever-present in his autobiography. What has changed between these two generations (and representations of two different class positions within two generations) is the rela-tionship of men to money. Put as boldly as this, the idea immedi-ately invites dissent and disagreement, in that the Grub Street of literature is as old as printing, and the financial gains of writ-ing have always been attractive. It is not argued here that this relationship has changed, or in any sense differed from one period to another during the twentieth century. It is the level of anxiety and concern which is at issue, and the way in which the greater social security of Orwell and Waugh made these writers more detached, although no less concerned, about money. Larkin, for example, writes in a way which suggests precisely that psychic permeation by the cash nexus which Marx argued was one of the consequences of capitalism. The famous 'cut price crowd' of Larkin's poetry is echoed throughout his letters by an endless concern with the financial costs of both material objects and, more tellingly, human relationships. A letter to his companion Monica Jones is typical of Larkin's organisation of personal and financial life. In the letter Larkin allows the financial generosity of Monica Jones and then immediately removes it by pointing to his own, meanly calculated largesse:

> The shock of parting from you . . . after a fortnight's close association, is sharp, leaving me feeling rather dull and indifferent. But I feel I can tell people I had a good holiday – putting up at swagger hotels in beautiful scenery with a lovely women eatin' and drinkin' my head off, I bet they'd envy me if they knew . . . Thank you dear for all your kindness and tolerance and beautiful behaviour, like buying me mint cake and the flannel. I'm not sure you weren't a bit out of pocket on the final deal: perhaps not, as I call the petrol 5/6d a gallon and said we got 30 miles for it, both errors in the right direction, though small ones.[39]

In all his dealings with the world, but most tellingly with women, Larkin assesses the financial cost of the contact and the engagement. As Larkin said in one of his more furious letters to Kingsley Amis: 'Everything about the ree-lay-shun-ship between men and women makes me *angry*.'[40]

Larkin continued to be angry for the rest of his life. Although he was capable of the most sustained courtesy towards women (as his letters and accounts of his visits to Barbara Pym demonstrate), he was also like Osborne, consistently unable to contain a fury at the desire he felt for women and could not adequately express. This constant protest about ambiguous feelings – of love and hate for women and attraction for and repulsion by them – is a theme that runs throughout Osborne and Larkin and can be read as more than individual pathology. Thus we can observe that both Larkin and Osborne acquired an early unease with their social roots and social origins: the authors of both *The Whitsun Weddings* and *Look Back in Anger* articulated an endless fury at the cultural domination of the bourgeois world. Inevitably, both writers were initially read as radicals (Osborne's own early associations with the Campaign for Nuclear Disarmament encompassed this reading). But inevitably the envy of both writers at a world, or worlds, which seems to exclude them became more marked. Both became, in different ways, Establishment figures; but Larkin in particular did much to associate himself not with the conservative politics of Macmillan and Home but, significantly, with the more socially radical politics of Margaret Thatcher. Larkin and Osborne became, by the end of their lives, convinced and vocal anti-modernists and in political terms, determined conservatives.

From a discussion of four figures – Orwell, Waugh, Larkin and Osborne – it is impossible to advance anything other than tentative interpretations about masculinity and the project of auto/biography. Of the four writers, all, with the exception of John Osborne, have been the subject of extensive biographical work, and all have in various ways been absorbed and integrated into the canon of English literature. The similarities between them, however, go further than merely the amount of attention paid to them by others. Two characteristics are particularly striking: their ambiguous relationship to sexuality (and their own sexuality in particular), and their terror of the world which they construct as either suburban or lower middle-class. The fear of the 'mass' therefore unites the authors of *Look Back in Anger* and *Brideshead Revisited*; these authors have no affection for the day-to-day experience of commonplace lives, not for them the delights of the *Diary of a Nobody's* Mr Pooter or the routines of family existence. Indeed, those general experiences of the majority of their compatriots (family life and community associations) are treated either satirically or as part of a different, inferior way of life. The adjectives 'smug' and 'boring' occur endlessly in their descriptions of everyday life, and Cyril Connolly's comment about 'the pram in the hall' being the end of artistic and/or intellectual aspirations is tacitly endorsed by all these authors.

What we can see in this pattern of terror about the incursions of domesticity is both the fear of men about the threat posed by domestic life to their sense of masculine identity and a last, frantic grasp at the ideal of the autonomous male hero. Both Waugh and Orwell undertook quasi-heroic adventures (Waugh in his days as a war correspondent and through foreign travel, and Orwell in military combat), while Larkin and Osborne used a model of the isolated, autonomous hero as the ideal of themselves. Relationships with women, as far as Larkin and Osborne are concerned, are about avoiding the sense of entrapment, of asserting individuality and, of course, endlessly maintaining separation. In this latter case, intimacy for these men is always problematic, since its very nature implies and involves the loss of self and the recognition of another person. Thus the project of masculine identity, for all these authors, is organised around their implicit protest at the ambiguity of masculinity. That femininity is equally ambiguous is seldom recognised: Osborne reserves his greatest hostility for women who are successful in conventional, careerist terms, while Larkin conscientiously avoided women who might in any way challenge the limits of his masculinity.

Being a man (and not being a woman) therefore consistently dominates the lives of these great writers of twentieth-century Britain. In the same generation, Jan (formerly James) Morris found the condition of masculinity impossibly burdensome. Through painful surgery and medical intervention, he became a woman. The same culture of sexual conformity which dominated – in an unspoken way – the lives of Orwell *et al.* resulted in Morris's (literal) transformation from man to woman. Morris's account of the reasons for, and consequences of, his decision to alter his gender identity are given in *Conundrum*.[41] In the review of the transition from man to woman, Morris makes it plain that he is aware of many of the issues which surround his decision, and in particular the futility of using the body, and alterations to the body, as a way of changing individual experiences of the world. As Morris writes: 'Would any conflict have been so bitter if I had been born now, when the gender line is so much less rigid? If society had allowed me to live in the gender I preferred, would I have bothered to change sex?'[42] But bother he does, and as a result:

> Psychologically I was distinctly less forceful. A neurotic condition common among women is called penis envy, its victims supposing that there is inherent to the very fact of the male organs some potent energy of the spirit. There is something to this fancy. It is not merely the loss of androgens that has made me more retiring, more ready to be led, more passive: the removal of the organs themselves has contributed, for there was to the presence of the penis something positive and stimulating. My body then was made to push and initiate, it is made now to yield and accept, and the outside change has had its inner consequences.[43]

Conundrum was first published in 1974, and the childhood and adolescence which Morris describes all took place during and just after the Second World War. As such, Jan Morris belongs to a younger generation than Waugh and Orwell, whose youth was lived before the Second World War, but to recognisably the same generation as Larkin and Osborne. Yet what is interesting about the various interpretations and manifestations of masculinity in this period (approximately 1920–60) is the greater affection (or at least toleration) for women and femininity in the older generation than the younger. Like Morris, Orwell and Waugh were drawn to what Waugh called 'soldiering'. Morris, in fact, spends some time in *Conundrum* praising what he describes as his 'beloved army'. We have seen that Morris's affection for women, and the state of femininity, is such that James is transformed into Jan. It is, of course, impossible to generalise about entire generations on the basis of individual cases, but what these cases do suggest is that diversity and difference in gender identity are long-standing cultural themes, and that the intolerance of femininity, homosexuality and gender instability, which so characterise the work of Larkin and Osborne, are part of a post-war culture: of late rather than early modernism.

This relationship between the construction of masculinity and modernism is a crucial one, in that we can see in it both the origins of that burden of masculinity which Morris felt determined to shed, and the inevitable crisis that masculinity was to encounter in the late twentieth-century West. The age in which Waugh and Orwell lived is chronologically close to that of Larkin and Osborne, but the meaning of the symbols of masculinity – in particular an association with the military – had changed dramatically after the Second World War. Waugh and Orwell belonged to a generation in which it was still possible for masculine military vigour and engagement to be seen as positive. For the Western powers the Second World War was a 'just' war, in which a specific form of masculinity – armed aggression – had a legitimate and valued place in the culture. Orwell, of course, was doubly involved in war and militarism: after his early employment in the Burmese colonial police, he fought for the Republican Army in Spain and a cause identified with democracy, progress and liberty. Yet after the Second World War the military lost its general legitimacy. Colonel Blimp was actually invented in the Second World War, and with that comic invention came a rejection not just of the military *per se*, but of military hierarchy. As Britain's military engagements changed after the Second World War, from a defence of democracy and a war against fascism to a battle for the empire, so the army became involved in campaigns that were increasingly seen as unacceptable. Of its place in the world during the years of the 1950s, Jan Morris wrote that 'I was activating impotence.'[44]

That quotation, and that comment on a particular aspect of individual biography, is extraordinarily evocative and suggestive with regard to the transformation of post-war culture, and the particular transformation of masculinity. Morris makes the comment in the light of an account of her professional successes, all of which are associated with maleness. ('I thought of public success itself, I suppose, as part of maleness, and I deliberately turned my back on it, as I set my face against manhood.')[45] What is apparent from this view is that a particularly successful person, in conventional terms, could not accept the assumptive world which went with the success achieved and made possible through orthodox masculinity. As Morris discovered, being successful was not a matter of achieving any absolute standard, but achieving distinction in relation to certain very fixed and rigid standards. A part of those standards was a construction of how to be male, and (although Morris is less emphatic on these points) white and middle-class as well. Clearly, what is recognised is that the nature of success, for individuals such as Morris, depends upon a certain acceptance of given hierarchies and, perhaps most importantly, the acceptance of privilege.

Much of *Conundrum* is given to the description of Jan Morris's feelings on the loss of the privileges of middle-class masculinity. For Philip Larkin and John Osborne the privileges of the middle-class world were not theirs to give up. Although Philip Larkin was born into a middle-class home and educated at Oxford, his experience of the world was confined to a particularly limited stratum of English provincial life; he was cosmopolitan in the associations of his education but narrow in his political and social experience. Osborne like Larkin, spent much of his life in one milieu, and again like Larkin had a deep distrust of the world outside Britain. As mass communication brought about a 'global' consciousness of world events, so Larkin and Osborne confined their lives increasingly to the British isles. The masculinity which Morris literally gave up never had the same positive associations for Larkin and Osborne; they did not relish in the glory of the military, of foreign travel and the easy superiority of the British ruling class. For them, all these possibilities were for various reasons denied, and their literal and metaphorical engagement with masculinity was more involved in battles with fictional armies of women than with the untutored hordes of the empire. In all, therefore it was not just the real possibilities of masculinity that changed after the Second World War but the fictional and fantastical possibilities as well. The military which had once been a defender of liberty became a defender of white imperial privilege, and as that transformation occurred so it left a considerable vacuum in the ways in which masculinity could be constructed. Financial and intellectual success were possible, but British culture had never enthusiastically endorsed either. (Waugh's character Rex Mottram in *Brideshead Revisited* stands as a definitive example of the stupidity of the financially successful.)

In this post-war world, therefore, the biographical (not to mention autobiographical) options open to men both changed, and in certain ways decreased. In the 1960s the emergence of a popular youth culture was to offer models of success in entertainment, but the discontent of Osborne's Jimmy Porter was rooted in a culture that was both older and specifically British. Like his close friend Kingsley Amis, Larkin turned to an angry and misogynistic rant against the twentieth century: women, the working class, youth culture and Labour governments were all to blame for the disappearance of a secure world. As the world in many ways became a more predictable world for women (in that contraception made possible the control of fertility, and a diminishing belief in patriarchal authority opened up the restrictions of family life), so it inevitably became less secure for men.

Jan Morris took, therefore, the radical step of leaving what s/he seems to have perceived as a threatened tribe before it finally became extinct. To men like Osborne and Larkin, who did not choose this route, the construction of themselves involved not an identification with potent symbols of masculinity, but a resistance to those aspects of modernism (notably the feminine and the cosmopolitan) that seemed particularly threatening. Nevertheless, both made considerable, distinguished careers out of opposition and resistance to modernity. Osborne's biography remains to be written, but in writing that of Philip Larkin,

Andrew Motion reminded his readers that Larkin himself was distrustful of the basic tenets of biography:

> Larkin liked to scoff at many of the basic tenets of biography itself. He divided its willingness to rely for psychological insights on formative childhood experiences. 'Whenever I read an autobiography', he said, 'I tend to start halfway through, when the chap's grown up and it becomes interesting.' In the same way, he repudiated the idea that writers might evolve in response to what happened to them in adult life. 'Only mediocrities develop,' he was fond of saying, quoting Oscar Wilde.[46]

Larkin is well known for having scoffed endlessly at his prospective biographer, Jake Balokowsky, but when Motion came to take on the role in real life he found that Larkin had prepared the way for a biographer by the accumulation of an extensive and thorough archive of his life. Biography clearly was not to be entirely rejected, even if Larkin himself regarded, as the passage above indicates, the origins of the person (the 'chap' in this case) with less than interest. We can also read in that absence of interest a rejection of the domestic world; when 'chaps' grow up they generally leave home and their mothers, and enter the world of adult men. For avowedly heterosexual men, such as Larkin and Osborne, the world of childhood is a place, in part, of fear and loathing, since it is the place in which they may not be able to escape from female control and dominance. Today, therefore, it is possible to suggest that autobiography and biography by and of men contains not just the obvious and conventional problems of transformation within a genre, but a more fundamental problem of how to locate the masculine in relationship to the person and the subjective self. For women, the self has always been assumed to be less unitary, and more private. The extent to which it is also dominated by a search for a hero is, however, the theme of the following chapter.

Chapter 5

Looking for daddy

The relationship between masculinity, autobiography and the twentieth century is inevitably complicated by questions about the nature of modernity, and the relationship of masculinity to cultural shifts and changes of pre- and post-Holocaust Europe. The 'hero' of the nineteenth-century empire clearly changes, in the twentieth century, into a less immediately authoritarian and hierarchical figure. Yet heroes persist, and the coincidence of the defence of Western liberalism with the soldier hero of the Second World War is a very powerful one. At the same time, we can observe that, at least in British culture, the period between the First and Second World Wars was one in which – particularly in the writing of Virginia Woolf and the Auden group – the 'modern' was identified with a more diverse form of masculinity than had previously been allowed.[1] The identification of literacy and artistic sensibility with homosexuality became a very close one, and although it was vehemently resisted by writers such as Lawrence and Orwell, it was nevertheless part of a tradition of resistance to the muscular masculinity that had formed the ethos of the public schools, the military and imperial administration.

Thus not being part of this persona of masculinity was to a certain extent an act of political dissent. To refuse the uniform of masculinity (both literally and metaphorically) carried with it possibilities of other identifications: with the cerebral and the radical, and with the cosmopolitan and the secular. As with all identities, constructing a version of masculinity was complex, and related not just to gender but to class, age and race. Even if there were different versions of masculinity for different middle- and upper-class men, they still remained white and privileged. Refusing (as Orwell did) the badges of privileges did not necessarily imply that educated, middle-class Englishmen turned their back on the bourgeois world. Throughout the twentieth century we can therefore see that shifts in masculine identity were a constant theme of the culture; even though an emphasis on physical courage became problematic after the First World War, the valorisation of male physical strength remained consistent. Indeed, the male body as a sign, and signifier, of masculinity arguably became – in its various disguises of German fascism, Soviet Socialism, Bloomsbury aesthetic and Hollywood screen idols – more influential in the twentieth century than in any other. The influence of masculinity can equally be seen in the dress and the behaviour of women. Wearing trousers and choosing short haircuts became a fashion for women. Even in the feminised versions of masculinity (for example, such Hollywood figures as Katherine Hepburn and Joan Crawford), what was being adopted as dress by women was derived from male clothing.[2]

But just as we can identify considerable visual evidence of the diversity of the ideal of masculinity, it is also legitimate to ask about the ways in which the lived experience of masculinity became, in the twentieth century, more rather than less problematic. The gradual emancipation of women from a private space and from limited public agency raised questions about relations between the sexes which were first mooted in the 'new women' debates of the late nineteenth century and continued throughout the twentieth century.[3] Essentially, contraception and economic emancipation gave a material reality to the goal of the 'denaturalisation' of male/female relations which has long been a part of some Western agendas. Few nineteenth-century authors could escape from naturalistic assumptions about the 'essence of womanhood', but the technological changes produced by the twentieth century undermined the assumption of the inevitable divisions between the sexes. For women, this offered real opportunities for the transformation of personal relationships. For men, on the other hand, this emancipation (however limited and partial) destabilised certain assumptions about masculinity and produced, as autobiography and biography demonstrate, some degree of uncertainty about 'being' male.[4] Orwell, as we have seen, had to resort to sentimental versions of working-class life in order to find an acceptable version of masculinity. In the same generation, Waugh self-consciously and emphatically created for himself the life of a traditional patriarch in order to 'find' an assured and coherent version of masculinity. Indeed, despite their wide political differences, the two men shared a great deal in their resolution of masculine contradictions and ambiguities. Both had a certain respect for a military life, even if experience tempered, in both cases, their enthusiasm. Both retained respect and affection for the idea (if not the reality) of traditional family life, and both found it difficult to understand women in anything other than stereotypical ways.

Thus, from different positions within the political spectrum, and with different experiences of the twentieth century, these two men reveal a certain consistency in white, middle-class behaviour and attitudes. It is quite apparent from their writing that both retained the idea of a hero, and of the possibilities of entirely creditable action by male individuals. Men could, in the fiction of Waugh and Orwell, know and follow moral principles, and they could also act on these principles. Moreover, the principles were absolute and universal; not for either of them the possibilities of the moral uncertainties of modernity, in which multiple realities of experience can create a multiplicity of moral responses. What is maintained here, then, is a real and lived version of a single, universal morality, in which judgements are free from qualifications about situation and circumstance. It is precisely this kind of judgement and assumption that Carol Gilligan challenges in her book on moral judgement, *In a Different Voice*, and in doing so initiates a debate on moral judgement which remains influential.[5]

The importance of Gilligan, and others who have taken up

her work, is that she offers to women, and others outside the privileged enclosure of the white, male middle class, the possibility of a view of the world which is as equally valid and legitimate as that of the privileged. The crisis of masculinity in the late twentieth century West is not, therefore, a crisis about the disappearance of the social and political power of masculinity, but about its legitimacy. Waugh and Orwell wrote in a world that took for granted the possibility of achieving a shared view of that world; they did not agree, but they understood and recognised certain central values and assumptions which were, in a very real sense, not negotiable. But post-1945, those certainties disappear. They disappear with the recognition that it was those very certainties about the nature of thought and morality that made possible the Holocaust and the demise of the idea of moral progress implicit in the Enlightenment. Precisely because it was always men who were most centrally concerned with this project, so it was inevitable that men should be most affected by the loss of those moral certainties – or the possibility of the search for moral certainty – which earlier generations had taken for granted.

Hence writing about men, and writing the biography of men (or men writing their autobiography) has had to face, post-1945, the issue of the changed nature of the public space and the relationship of men to it. That secure mirror which the public space once offered to men, particularly in post-Enlightenment Europe, disappeared, and with it the model for the interpretation of lived experience. Women, who have always lived a more private life than men, could now speak with greater certainty precisely because their lives had changed relatively little. At the same time, the thesis of this chapter is that the disappearance of the orderly (or at least ordered) world of post-Enlightenment masculinity posed problems for women just as much for men. These were not problems of the same kind, but they were nevertheless substantial, in that women were now left with a world which had become free of iconographic masculinity. The personal, individual consequences of life without heroes for women is the concern of this discussion.

Two women – both authors of distinction and both authors of autobiography – who exemplify the problem for women of a world without the possibility of heroism are Germaine Greer and Sylvia Plath. From Australia and the United States respectively, they have acquired identification (albeit a problematic identification) with feminism and with issues related to women. Both, as is still apparent in the case of Germaine Greer, found identification with women deeply disturbing and constructed powerful accounts of the possibilities of female agency in order to solve, and resolve, the potential powerlessness of femininity. Yet in each the disappearance of the assurance of the male hero raised problems which structured the nature of their work.

In the case of Germaine Greer, there is considerable evidence to suggest that her entire *oeuvre* has been autobiographical. Indeed, as is the case of Simone de Beauvoir, Germaine Greer fully meets our expectations of an 'autobiographical' writer, in which the inevitable use of personal experience is extended well beyond the normal expectations of the writing of fiction. Greer's main themes, from the limits of female desire and the prescriptions about female agency that form the theme of *The Female Eunuch*, to the discussion about infertility and children which inspires *Sex and Destiny*, are clearly themes close to the author's own situation.[6] Nevertheless, these two works are presented as objective non-fiction, a categorisation which distinguishes them from Greer's *Daddy, We Hardly Knew You*, an explicitly autobiographical account of the author's search for the identity of her father.[7] Greer did not have to find a father in a literal sense, since Germaine Greer grew up with her father and he lived well in to her adult life, but she did have to discover who her father was, in the sense of acquiring information about his parenthood and his social origins. The father – not literally missing but metaphorically far from present – determines the search, and the subject, of the book. What emerges from Germaine Greer's account of her long and gruelling search for information about her father is that both father and daughter were deeply influenced by ideas about male heroism, about constructing a male life in terms that suggest engagement with the forces of evil and the emergence of a spectacular form of moral triumph. Ironically, the person who emerges from the book as the hero is not the deceitful and largely inadequate Mr Greer but his wife, Germaine Greer's mother. Despite the portrayal of this woman as silly and stupid, it is quite apparent that it was in fact Mrs Greer who bought up three children and maintained a home and normality.

But this contribution to her daughter's life is largely refused in *Daddy, We Hardly Knew You*. Thus what emerges from the book is that, even when the full extent of the father's inadequacy and deceit is unmasked by the daughter, it is still the mother, and the mother's part in the child's life, which is denied. The mother is ruthlessly described, held up for mockery and endlessly criticised: nowhere is the existence of three competent and in many ways successful children introduced as in any sense relevant to the *curriculum vitae* of Mrs Greer. The final chapter of *Daddy, We Hardly Knew You* leaves her, not as reconciled to her daughter or her husband's newly revealed past, but as a half-mad semi-vagrant:

> She was wearing a skin-tight synthetic knit dress, striped green, yellow and white. 'It's nice, isn't it?' she had said. 'I found it on a fence. Yes, somebody must have got wet, and it's awful to sit in a car in a sopping dress, so they took it off and left it on the fence. I found it when I was out on my bike. I find all sorts of things when I'm out on my bike.' She smoothed the dress over her hips, evidently quite satisfied with her own improbable theory about its provenance. 'Yes, no, yes, I'm a scavenger, a beach-comber. That's how I live.' I reflected that, to a woman who treated the whole world as a series of beaches, it was perfectly consistent to treat everything in it as flotsam and jetsam.[8]

What follows this account does not, in many ways, make comfortable reading. Mother and daughter bicker and jostle for conversational control. It is evident that Mrs Greer, unable to compete in terms of formal education and cosmopolitan experience with her daughter, talks back in a mode of fantasy and barbed comments on aspects of her famous daughter's biography. But what perhaps matters most here is the revelation of Germaine Greer's assumption that we, as readers, will take her side in the contest between mother and daughter. We are to be seduced by talk of the mad mother who steals clothes and makes unsuitable remarks about half-naked men. Seduction of the reader, is of course, not all that far from the daughter's attempted seduction of the father – a seduction which, in the case of Germaine Greer, was manifestly unsuccessful in that the father remained resolutely negative about his famous daughter. However, what we need to take from this chapter of *Daddy, We Hardly Knew You* are two aspects of Germaine Greer's autobiography. First, there is the assumption that the reader, the audience, occupies the same metaphorical space as the father; by implication, therefore, the audience is male and it is to be seduced by a determined logic and understanding of the world. Second, Germaine Greer articulates a distaste for what she perceives as the feminine (confused, incoherent, unsystematic), which puts her in a position not unlike that of John Osborne. Indeed, the mother of John Osborne appears almost as an identical twin to the mother of Germaine Greer – endlessly powerful, endlessly infuriating and apparently undermining of their children's activities.

Except, of course, that the undermining which the children perceive in their mother's behaviour is matched by the encouragement and the confidence that these children have received, and have clearly received from their mothers. Unless we accept whole-heartedly the rejection of theories about nurture and the importance of childhood experiences, we have to acknowledge that it is from their relationships with these mocked, despised (and very much feared) mothers that the authors of *Look Back in Anger* and *The Female Eunuch* acquired much of both their creativity and their imagination. One of the many ironies of the accounts by Germaine Greer and John Osborne of their mothers is that they attack them for their deceitfulness and refusal of what their children describe as reality. To their children these faults are unforgivable, yet as readers we can see that the other side to these qualities (or perhaps other names for these qualities) is an understanding of fantasy and an irreverence for the apparent rules and boundaries of the everyday world. In this light, we can read Mrs Greer's account of the origins of her dress not as her daughter does – which is that the account is a pack of lies – but as a piece of comic invention. Mrs Greer's story of her new dress suggests a rich vein of imagination: she makes up a person for her story, and tells a tale about her relationship to the dress.

But the voice of the law – as truth only understandable within the limits of the literal – denies the possibilities of this tale. What the child wanted, and what the adult Germaine Greer wanted, was a reliable version of the world, a masculine version of the world that could empower and allow a way out of the domestic fantasies of the female world. Mrs Greer's embroideries about the world did not fit well with the expectations of the formal, institutional world in which her daughter wished to do well. On the other hand, what she offered to her daughter was an acceptance of marginality:

> My mother had no class pretensions, no snobbery, no toffery. She was too eccentric to merge with the mass of suburban housewives. She watched no soap-opera, played no bridge, belonged to no women's organisation, worked for no charity, drank with no girlfriends ... There was something very unbourgeois and unworldly about this life-style, which I imagine emanated from my mother, who was perfectly happy to dress in hand-me-downs and cast-offs, supplemented by her own rather haphazard dress-making.[9]

This experience, this kind of childhood, was one which was seen as peculiar and eccentric. Indeed, Germaine Greer's account of it is that it was unhappy and lacking in the flowers, paintings and music which she describes in the same chapter as essential to the good life. But what she looks back on as loss, readers can see as functional to the thirst for education and wider horizons which eventually took her to Cambridge and the wide world. What Greer does not entertain is that, from our losses and our experience of absence, we can often learn to acquire the necessary compensation.

Throughout Germaine Greer's account of her childhood and her search for her father there is little to suggest that in the background, as a constant figure, was her mother. When Mrs Greer occasionally appears, she is portrayed as eccentric, abnormal, and above all threatening, the nightmare mother who meets her daughter's friends wearing underpants on her head. What she is, to her daughter is 'vain, capricious, manipulative, unreliable, girlish, affected, infantile'.[10] As her daughter goes on to say, '*The Female Eunuch* was not written.'[11] But when it was written, it was an act of revenge against her mother and as such joins other influential works by women that can be described as 'revenge literature'. Yet, while many of these works (including, for example, Sylvia Plath's *The Bell Jar*) are motivated by women's fury at the apparent hopelessness and impotence in which the feminine condition, and their mothers, imprisoned them, they also share another characteristic: they cannot avoid a male subject, even if the apparent subject is female. *Daddy, We Hardly Knew You* illustrates particularly clearly the difficulty that women face in writing autobiography. All genres of narrative literature (be they fiction or auto/biography) tend to be structured according to a relatively fixed pattern of gender development. This underlying plot structure is one in which the narrative agent (or hero) must be male, regardless of the actual person in the text, because the detours and obstacles that have to be overcome are morphologically female. Thus the overall 'plot' of culture, and literature in particular, is one in which men occupy the heroic space.

Mr Greer is thus the 'hero' of *Daddy, We Hardly Knew You*. But this example, while a particularly vivid example of the way in which women cannot avoid the gendered dynamic of narrative, is also particularly transparent in its presentation of the female/mother as difficulty and opposition and the male/father as the source of agency. The search for the identity of this agency constitutes the narrative of the book, but with it comes a resolution that shifts agency, and certainly the moral status of the hero, from the father to the social mother. When Germaine Greer discovers the 'good' mother (her father's foster mother) she discovers a form of mothering with which she can identify. What is important about this mothering is that it is chosen, deliberate and not biological: the 'real' mother is precisely not that, and as such represents a woman who was independent of the claims of the biological father. The multiple dedication of the book, 'to my three grandmothers' effectively undermines patriarchal identity and patriarchal control. In that sense, *Daddy, We Hardly Knew You* could be read as a work of feminist recovery, in which valiant and sympathetic women such as Mr Greer's foster mother are validated and rewarded. That reading is certainly acceptable as testimony to the care and concern of the women concerned.

But what that reading obscures, and ignores, is the complete disavowal – which amounts almost to a disowning – of the real mother. To praise unknown women, and to write hymns of praise about their tenacity and courage (even if those hymns have a basis in fact) is to choose between the reality of individual identity (the sad fate of maturing) and the fantastical identities beloved of children and the dispossessed. The real parents to whom Germaine Greer was born are both declared missing by the end of the book: the mother has no place in rational discourse, and the father has no place as a representative of truth or virtue. Lost in the same narrative is any sense of the mutual deceit of the parents: if Mr Greer invented his past, then his wife clearly colluded with it, even at the cost of her own hold on what her daughter sees as reality. Yet, just as the possibility of something called 'reality' is introduced into this account, so it is impossible not to notice that, for the daughter, the escape from the oppressive fantasies of her parents is into the equally fantastical world (and, it has to be said, the deeply gendered world) of English Literature. If there was no literal hero at home, then one had to be discovered on the library shelves.

Daddy, We Hardly Knew You is explicitly organised around a search for an individual hero. For other women writers of auto/biography in the twentieth century the search for a site of agency is organised around the same search for a hero (the first two volumes of Simone de Beauvoir's autobiography being just one example) or a search for a more general form of understanding and possible agency. Typical of the second form of sub-genre is Alice Kaplan's *French Lessons*, in which the author writes of her adolescent adoption of French as the language in which she could truly speak.[12] She writes of this:

> I can't imagine not having French. I think I would starve without it. Why do people want to adopt another culture? Because there's something in their own they don't like, that doesn't name them.
>
> French still calls out to me in the most primitive way. If I'm in a crowded room and there are two people speaking French all the way on the other side of the room, I'll hear, loud as day, as though a friend were calling my name. My ears prick up. I become all ears, hearing every word, noticing the words I don't know or haven't heard for a while and remembering when I last heard them. I'll eavesdrop shamelessly, my attention now completely on that conversation, as if I belong in it; I'll start trying to figure out how to get in on it.[13]

In this extract Alice Kaplan has illustrated two aspects of women's relationship to auto/biographical writing which have been widely commented on. The first is the relationship between the need (literally the hunger) to write or express oneself and the assumption of the psychic impulse to repair the damage of castration to the sense of the female self. Melanie Klein's writing on creativity and artistic agency has greatly illuminated the underlying motives that compel us to attempt to 'mend' the damage of the wound of castration, of not being male, by the creation of cultural products.[14] This hunger to create is precisely what Alice Kaplan speaks of when she speaks of 'starving' without French. But the other sense in which she would metaphorically 'starve' without French is in the sense of not having access to an alternative world, an alternative and much more feminine world of grace and pleasure, to that of the literal, factual world of her father, the lawyer. In a striking passage earlier in the book, Alice Kaplan writes of the experience of sharing a meal with her mother, a meal at which they both forget their individual problems in shared pleasure, a pleasure which is represented by France:

> It was hard to get my mother to eat without thinking of her ulcer, and I was still on my breadcrust diet, but France had gotten to both of us – its pleasure principle – and our separate abnegations had broken down in sync. The bouillabaisse involved a ritual of croutons, aioli, special thin forks for penetrating mussels, bibs to encourage carefree manners. We went at the bouillabaisse with total determination. She forgot she was sick; I forgot I was angry. We put away the whole pot.[15]

At this groaning French table, mother and daughter share pleasure; they both, as Alice Kaplan describes, forget their individual problems in the delight of food. France becomes the shared and 'good' external world, in which differences can be forgotten and the hunger created by phallic absence assuaged. Mother and daughter literally bond through food; as the infant was once fed by the mother, either literally or metaphorically, so they again feed in a way which is shared and healing.

Alice Kaplan is fortunate in that she finds a culture and its detail in which she can locate her sense of herself and her sense of difference from her father and her native United States. In this awareness of finding solace in exile she shares exactly the same biographical position as Sylvia Plath and Germaine Greer – great female voices of the twentieth century who have to leave home and country in order to find cultures where they can express their sense of themselves. Plath's departure for England and Cambridge after she graduated from Smith College in Massachussetts took her to a world in which she could place herself, both geographically and socially, at a distance from her mother's suburban aspirations and reality. In *The Bell Jar*, written years after her arrival in England and after her marriage to Ted Hughes and the birth of her children, Sylvia Plath could clearly still remember her fierce hatred for the Eisenhower version of the good American life. Despite the antagonism which Plath often expressed towards England and its inhabitants (its cold, its dirt and its class structure), she nevertheless found in exile the circumstances in which she could write and avoid the perceived pressures to conform to a narrow version of reality. That narrow construction of reality is what Plath describes as 'the motherly breath of the suburbs', which 'smelt of lawn sprinklers and station-wagons and tennis rackets and dogs and babies!'[16] It is a marginally more prosperous world than that of Germaine Greer's family home, but the aspirations and the culture are the same; they form part of that suburban world which was being exported by the United States in the 1950s as the admirable, definitive way of life.

But what *The Bell Jar* recognises so well is that the implicit contract of that suburban life-style is one which assumes the dependence of women and the rule of patriarchy in the home. Fantasising about life in this world, Sylvia Plath wrote:

> I tried to imagine what it would be like if Constantin were my husband. It would mean getting up at seven and cooking him eggs and bacon and toast and coffee and dawdling about in my nightgown and curlers after he'd left for work to wash up the dirty plates and make the bed, and then when he came home after a lively, fascinating day he'd expect a big

dinner, and I'd spend the evening washing up even more
dirty plates till I fell into bed, utterly exhausted.

This seemed a dreary and wasted life for a girl with fifteen
years of straight A's, but I knew that's what marriage was
like, because cook and clean and wash was just what Buddy
Willard's mother did from morning till night, and she was
the wife of a university professor and had been a private
school teacher herself.[17]

The Sylvia Plath/Esther Greenwood character in *The Bell Jar*
opts out of this ideal both by rejecting Buddy Willard and then
by attempting suicide. The contrast between the account of this
adolescence (a barely disguised account of Sylvia Plath's own life)
and that of Germaine Greer in the suburbs of Melbourne is that,
while Mrs Plath did everything she could to integrate herself
(and her family) into the narrative structure of the 1950s in the
United States, Mrs Greer was quite content, as her daughter
bitterly pointed out, to turn her back on all expectations of good
housekeeping and pretensions about the home beautiful. At the
same time it is apparent from *Daddy, We Hardly Knew You* that
Germaine Greer longed for a more fully realised version of the
domestic ideal, although as readers we can see that Mrs Greer,
unlike the self-sacrificing Mrs Plath, was bent on a career of what
has become known, and read, as resistance. The Mrs Plaths (or
more particularly the Mrs Willards) who spent their lives trying to
live up to the standards and expectations of the 1950s were to be
found, by Betty Friedan, going slowly crazy in this false promise
of paradise. *The Feminine Mystique*, published in 1963, offered a
message of hope to the Mrs Willards of the West: the fault is not
in you if you cannot accept this life, it is in the social system
which has constructed this version of the good life.[18]

When Sylvia Plath wrote *The Bell Jar* she had cut her ties with
the suburban life-style in which she had been brought up and was
living in England with her husband and two children. Yet for all
that literal emancipation (and physical distance between that culture and her mother), it is apparent from her letters to her

mother and her poetry that she was still deeply involved in the habits of the culture from which she had apparently escaped. The good housewife still cooked and cleaned and sent home reports of domestic competence and good behaviour. The punishing demands and expectations of domesticity were still an ever-present part of her existence, and ones which testify to the strength of the culture which produced them. It is that cultural strength and dominance of domesticity which other women writing about the 1950s have observed. Growing up in England, Carolyn Steedman observed her mother struggling against the stigma of being a woman with two 'illegitimate' children, and writes, 'The home was full of her terrible tiredness and her terrible resentment; and I knew it was all my fault.'[19]

We know, and Carolyn Steedman knows, that it was not in any way her 'fault'. The fault lay with an oppressive moral and social code which legitimated male heterosexuality while it assumed female economic and moral dependence. To be a 'good woman' you had to accept both sets of male assumptions about the world: the code which assumed male heterosexual desire and the code which assumed female responsibility for male morality. Sylvia Plath's disgust at Buddy Willard's double standard of sexual morality was a disgust echoed by generations of women who had to accept a male sense of heterosexual entitlement. Thus these angry accounts of the 1950s by Greer, Plath and by Steedman all speak of the damage done to the lives of individual women by the dominant sexual mores. As Valerie Walkerdine and Helen Lucey write at the beginning of *Democracy in the Kitchen: Regulating Mothers and Socialising Daughters*:

> When John Osborne looked back in anger in the 1950s, what he saw was the kitchen sink. The focus of his anger was a working-class kitchen, with a mother leading a stultifying life. The working-class grammar-school boys who at that time inaugurated the genre of realist kitchen-sink drama deeply despised their class. They especially hated their mothers with their piles of ironing and lack of conversation.

By contrast, other men who grew up in those times eulogised
their mothers, as Carolyn Steedman has so clearly remarked
about the writing of, for example, Richard Hoggart and
Jeremy Seabrook.[20]

This quotation provides a reminder that accounts of the past,
and family life, are deeply (and very specifically) gendered. But at
the same time the quotation also suggests some ways in which the
fate which Greer and Plath railed against (that is, to be like their
mothers) was also derided and loathed by many men. Osborne,
Larkin and Amis longed for apparently undomesticated women
and fantasised about women living lives unlike those of their
mothers. Thus a generation of women and men came together
in a protest against a domestic role for women, but it was a
protest which, perhaps inevitably, was weighted towards male
interests. Hence Greer marginalises and satirises her mother (and
her mother's resistance), while Plath took the path of absolute,
and finally destructive, identification with a male other. Feminists
have often written of Ted Hughes's brutality and callous cruelty
to Plath, but the other side of that particular marriage was the
heavy weight of expectation which Hughes was assigned.[21] The
evisceration of men in the cause of masculinity (against which
male writers have long protested) meant that women could not
find in men the sympathy they desired. As repressing the need for
intimacy with others became a taken-for-granted characteristic
of masculinity, so the escape *to* men proved deeply unsatisfying
for women.

But locked into these social and emotional expectations there
was nowhere for Plath and Greer (or Larkin and Osborne) to go.
The women endlessly disappointed Larkin and Osborne, since
they either seemed to present another version of maternal dominance or, in refusing that model, had no emotional resonance.
Plath and Greer desperately wanted to find male strength and
male answers in the academic and intellectual world that could
provide what was perceived as emancipation and liberation from
the bonds, both literal and metaphorical, of the household and

the feminine. In this deadly collusion both masculinity and femininity failed, and could do nothing except fail, since both were built on fantasies that had little relationship to the complexity and essential ambiguity of human existence. Those ambiguities are not, as Carolyn Steedman so elegantly demonstrates, only ambiguities of personal identity, they are also ambiguities about class and status. The British class system (even when internalised by 'outsiders' such as Greer and Plath) was sufficient to create an unhappy negotiation between class and gender, in which women were often forced to identify with a masculine symbolic and intellectual order to escape from the over-determinations of femininity and consequent absence of agency.

Acquiring agency – not the 'getting of wisdom' but the getting of agency – dominates women's biographical and autobiographical writing in the twentieth century. It is, of course, the other side of the coin to constructions of male heroism and implicit agency, and part of the irony of the gender relations of twentieth-century auto/biography is that, just as many men, from Lytton Strachey to Sartre, were questioning the prescribed order of aggressive masculinity, so women were asserting a right to autonomy and independence which matched every ideal of the heroic. The language of the literature of twentieth-century suffrage movements, on both sides of the Atlantic, is replete with a vocabulary of war and confrontation – the 'struggle', the 'cause' and the 'fight' are the terms in which campaigns are organised and presented. The legacy of this language, and more importantly the conceptual understanding implicit in it, is that any argument or any attempt to shift the position of women tends to be positioned within a rhetoric of male versus female, masculinity versus femininity. The more usual relationship between women and men in which collusion, if not co-operation, constitutes a major part of the engagement is lost in an understanding that cannot escape from the deadly domain of a particular form of agency as the definitive form of human action. Heroism, and its expectation, thus distorts the behaviour of both women and men. Women seek strength outside themselves (*à la* de Beauvoir or Plath). In doing so they invest strength in male others and construct the sense of omnipotence and entitlement which then destroys both relationships and, often, the heroes that have been created. Plath's poem 'Daddy' has always been read as the definitive female rejection of masculinity of the twentieth century, but it is also a poem, as Jacqueline Rose points out, which allows a second reading in which women are involved in the construction not just of brutality, but of fascism as well. Rose writes: 'In its most notorious statement, the poem suggests that victimisation by this feared and desired father is one of the fantasies at the heart of fascism, one of the universal attractions for women of fascism itself. As much as predicament, victimisation is also pull.'[22]

In the case of Sylvia Plath, the male other destroyed (at least symbolically) by over-investment in his strength was Ted Hughes: he became the fallen god in Plath's construction of her auto/biography. As Janet Malcolm has suggested in *The Silent Woman* (a study of biography and biographers of Sylvia Plath which is also subtitled 'Sylvia Plath and Ted Hughes'), the potential understanding of the life of Sylvia Plath was heavily over-determined, on all sides, by the different agendas that different individuals brought to their subject.[23] To a very considerable extent, *The Silent Woman* is an argument for the impossibility of biography, and at the same time as Janet Malcolm is arguing this case, she is also admitting to sympathies for Ted Hughes and his sister and against, if not Sylvia Plath, then her sympathetic biographers. She writes: 'As the reader knows, I, too have taken a side – that of the Hugheses and Anne Stevenson – and I, too, draw on my sympathies and antipathies and experiences to support it. But in the Plath–Hughes debate my sympathies are with the Hugheses.'[24] Thus we have a position which suggests on the one hand the impossibility of biography (not a new theme to Janet Malcolm) in the conventionally understood sense of a definitive account of a life, and on the other a sympathy for a particular interpretation of that life which has to depend on a view, a position, about it. Janet Malcolm fully admits she is partisan, but her partisanship is as much related to the biographers of Hughes and Plath as to the subject themselves.

In terms of Janet Malcolm's position in the discussion of Sylvia Plath, it is understandable that she should see Sylvia Plath as the first person who deliberately misunderstood her own biography and wilfully took revenge on those people – particularly her mother – whom she felt had tormented her or in some way served her badly. In chronological terms this argument is accurate, since it was the publication of *The Bell Jar* which encouraged Sylvia's mother to publish *Letters Home* (the correspondence between Sylvia and her mother), which in turn released endless comment and speculation about all the characters (including Mrs Plath) in the drama. This reading is, of course, dangerously close to the blame-the-victim accounts of women's oppression that have been widely attacked in feminist literature. Malcolm's case – that the controversy about Plath begins with Plath herself – invites us to judge Plath as vengeful and destructive, a woman set on the destruction of those people who tried to help her when she was most vulnerable.

But whether or not Sylvia Plath (or Ted Hughes, Olwyn Hughes, or any of the other main characters in the saga of the literature on Plath) emerges as the heroine or the villain is, in this context, beside the point. The lesson to be drawn from the furious and bitter controversy about readings and interpretations of Sylvia Plath is that many critics will go to great lengths to avoid general themes in biography and accept only explanations that prioritise individual pathology. In *The Silent Women* all the protagonists, with the exception of Ted Hughes who never appears in person, are in some way presented as pathological. That we all possess a degree of pathology is one thing, but Janet Malcolm gives to Anne Stevenson, Olwyn Hughes *et al.* formidable amounts of the pathological. Yet what is not suggested is that the devotion of all these individuals to the life of a dead person is in itself pathological; the person in the case is indeed compellingly interesting, but what kind of boundaries are being crossed between acceptable interest and compulsive voyeurism is a question which might be asked. Since the question is not asked, a biography of Sylvia Plath becomes impossible, in that no biographer is willing to allow either that the person is unknowable or that biographers project their own fantasies and needs on to their subjects.

What emerges from the literature, biographical and auto-biographical, about Sylvia Plath is that writers on the subject approach their central character with deeply partisan feelings. Thus accounts of Plath's life become arguments for particular intellectual positions, obviously grounded in the details of Plath's biography but with a politics and an understanding derived from elsewhere. Hence the case of Plath suggests both the refusal of the limits of biography (that it can ever be 'objective' or accurate in anything other than strictly factual terms) and the refusal of theoretical understandings which suggest that individuals share common needs and interests. This, in the case of Plath, would allow that she, like millions of other women, wanted a hero for a husband, and that the hopes invested on that hero limited the likely success of a real marriage. The strength of individuality, and individualism, in Western culture is, however, such that allowing these themes is often unacceptable. Writing about themselves and about others, women, have consistently found it difficult to come to terms with their collusion with heroism. That collusion has in turn distracted biographers from the real person – who lived in a shared culture – to the unreal person who lived only in a world invented by themselves. Exceptional talents are one thing, exceptional circumstances are another. But the belief in them is central to the art of biography, and to the fantasy that individuals live lives which are separate both from general patterns in any culture and from other human beings. How to 'separate' is a crucial *rite de passage* for all human beings, yet for many auto/biographical writers that reality is consistently ignored in favour of its refusal. Men, as Chapter 4 suggested, do not easily separate from their mothers. Nor, it would seem, do women. But for women the nature of separation has to be constructed within a discourse which emphasises an achieved (if mythical) identity with men. The accounts of individual lives which emerge from these constructions are then, more often than not, fantasies in themselves. 'Real' lives are not lived in the pages of auto/biography.

Chapter 6

The imagined self:

The impossibility of auto/biography

Although in the Thatcherite decades in Britain the cliché 'I blame the government' became a single-factor analysis of all social ills, it is difficult to isolate one factor as inspiring auto/biography. We can note that it is a literary genre rather more beloved of Protestant countries than those where Roman Catholicism is the dominant religion, and that the great popularity of auto/biography with the book-buying public is largely a twentieth-century phenomenon. But at the same time we can note that all literary genres have acquired larger publics in the twentieth century, as advances in mass literacy and material wealth made book-buying a possibility for larger numbers of people. Equally, Roman Catholicism was, until recently, associated in Europe with relative poverty: it is only since the Second World War that the material, if not the cultural, differences between Protestant and Catholic Europe have begun to disappear.

Tempting as it is to blame Protestantism for many of the cultural ills of the twentieth century, it is nevertheless not an entirely convincing case. Equally, arguing that capitalism is to blame, in that it reduces all social relationships to commodities and the *diktat* of the market, does not significantly advance the argument, since we have been living in a capitalist society since the seventeenth century, and on it can be blamed virtually all social and material events. Capitalism, without any doubt, has provided the context in which writers have lived and worked, but since the difference between them extends from Jane Austen to Martin Amis and from Lytton Strachey to Andrew Morton, the explanatory use of capitalism as a single-factor explanation has to be limited. However, if we begin to put together just two of the factors mentioned here – capitalism and Protestantism – we begin to edge slightly closer to an understanding of the world which might allow us to understand the popularity of auto/biography with the book-buying public and the enthusiasm of authors for writing it.

Thus the argument I wish to advance here is that what auto/biography does is to offer us a chance to stabilise the uncertainties of existence. In many ways, for many people, existence in the twentieth century, at least in Europe, has acquired a remarkable, and contradictory, dualism. On the one hand, material existence has become more reliable: we can generally control fertility and the production of food. 'Nature', in the sense of the hitherto 'uncontrolled' order of the natural world, is thus no longer the apparently cruel and arbitrary power that it was in early nineteenth-century life. Women no longer, or very seldom, die in childbirth, and parents can expect to see their children live to adulthood. New patterns and processes of food distribution and production ensure that mass starvation is no longer a European experience. But at the same time as these new conditions of existence have appeared, Europe has in the last one hundred years lived through two land wars and the Holocaust. That mass starvation which was so confidently assumed to have disappeared just two sentences ago occurred in the Netherlands at the end of the Second World War, and in that same country nature, in the form of the North Sea, is still capable of wreaking havoc. So the apparent stability and plenty which many people can take for granted is accompanied by the knowledge that these conditions can change. E.J. Hobsbawm in his *The Age of Extremes* has noted the 'hunger for a secure identity' which he sees as a characteristic of the age. In his discussion of the twentieth century he quotes the German scientist Max Planck, who wrote in 1933 that:

We are living in a very singular moment of history. It is a moment of crisis in the literal sense of that word. In every branch of our spiritual and material civilisation we seem to have arrived at a critical turning point. This spirit shows itself not only in the actual state of public affairs, but also in the general attitude towards fundamental values in personal and social life . . . Now the iconoclast has invaded the temple of science. There is scarcely a scientific axiom that is not nowadays denied by somebody. And at the same time almost any nonsensical theory would be almost sure to find believers and disciples somewhere or other.[1]

Scarcely was the ink dry on Max Planck's paper when Hitler came to power. The definitively 'nonsensical' theory of the twentieth century, German fascism, was about to plunge Europe, and indeed much of the world, into war. But Planck, Hobsbawm, and indeed many other writers on the twentieth century, want us to reflect not merely on the horrors of the Holocaust and fascism, but also on the contrast these events offered to the apparent reason and rationality of the twentieth century. Much of the literature on the Holocaust highlights this contrast: on the one side the advances in science and social understanding (and social engineering) and on the other the plunge – but an orderly and rational plunge – into the dark night of Nazism.[2] Diverse writers have pointed out that the Holocaust was a child of the Enlightenment, perhaps not the favoured child but certainly closely identifiable with those ideas of order and orderliness bequeathed by rational pragmatism. Little wonder that, for many European citizens of the twentieth century, the dominant crisis of social existence was how to maintain a degree of human authenticity and spontaneity in the face of coercive social expectations about the nature of acceptable behaviour.

In the light of these dualistic expectations, it is hardly surprising that a literature developed which identified the form of twentieth-century society as deeply controlling, and controlled. From H.G. Wells to Aldous Huxley and George Orwell, a fiction emerged which expressed concern and horror at developments in social organisation. At the same time as Planck was writing, social science in the United States was beginning to develop a critique of 'mass' society, a critique which was to be much enhanced by German-Jewish intellectuals fleeing from the new order of Hitler's Germany.[3] In theory and in practice individuals throughout what can be described as 'the West' began to identify with the problems resulting from the apparent triumph of reason and state commitment to planning. The Soviet Union was seen, by sections of the Western left, as the society that was the child of ideals of rationality; a view that took little account of the brutality involved in bringing that society into being, and that marginalised or overlooked the more convincing association between the construction of the United States and the Enlightenment. 'Planning' became the required form for 'modern' societies, and the first years of the twentieth century saw a general commitment to its possibilities.

That 'the dream failed' is a well-known fact of European and indeed world history. More precisely what failed (or could not succeed, given the global context of a capitalist market) was centralised state planning, conducted either by the political left or the political right. But even to use the term 'fail' somehow suggests that there is a blueprint for social and political successes to which societies can aspire. There is no such blueprint, and the 'failure' has to be understood in terms of the inability of different regimes to fulfil different promises. Even so, state planning (whatever its political focus) did achieve some spectacular successes: whether in the alleviation of mass starvation (and mass illiteracy) in China and the old Soviet Union, or in the more limited social intervention of the Roosevelt administration in the United States, the achievements were real and identifiable. But these successes, significant in terms of individual lives, have to be set against the perception and understanding of planning that gained currency in the West. Crucial to the negative construction of planning were Orwell's *Animal Farm* and *1984*; both published after the Second World War, they gave support to those who saw in centralised planning some inevitable form of attack on human freedom. The novels took up the themes raised in the 1930s by Aldous Huxley in *Brave New World* and by Chaplin in *Modern Times*. Both novel and film suggest that the dominating characteristic of the modern world is the control of people by science and machines. Specifically scientific and technological rationality became feared as the carriers of anti-humanism.

In these years, and in the years after the Second World War, and after Hiroshima, when the powers of technology became apparent, the self and the person acquired a new uncertainty. No age has seen the absence of uncertainty, but the late twentieth century created its distinct kind of uncertainty, in that the potential of human scientific and 'rational' enquiry seemed to lack corresponding moral development. 'Progress' and 'reason' now had perjorative as well as positive meanings, and the very moral certainties that had appeared to make auto/biography as straightforward a matter as the 'good' life of reality were no longer present. Lytton Strachey absolutely understood the essential ambiguity of person which is a characteristic of all existence, but against his understanding we can set legions of twentieth-century auto/biographies which have attempted to achieve coherence in their presentation of the self.

The form of auto/biography carries with it some considerable responsibility for allowing authors to convey the impression that lives are lived in orderly and coherent ways. Thus what has to be recognised in any account of auto/biography is the collusion, whether conscious or not, between writers of auto/biography and the deep desire of late twentieth-century society for order and stability. The idea of the achievement of certainty is a deeply attractive one to Western society; without it, the prospect is raised that individuals live their lives in terms of a response to irrational needs and desires. What Marion Milner, in one of the most evocative titles in psychoanalytic literature, has called *The Suppressed Madness of Sane Men*, is the possibility that although much is predictable about human existence in social terms, other aspects of existence do not lend themselves so easily to confident prediction.[4] We know, for example, that the children (especially the male children) of middle-class professionals are likely to become middle-class professionals themselves, but we do not know why individual emotional biographies should be so varied and so complex.

But because auto/biography is almost always organised in terms of chronology, the narrative has an implicit structure which organises content in a way that can marginalise or ignore significant aspects of individual experience. Here, the most glaring examples are those auto/biographies written by men about 'great' public men in which childhood is given almost no discussion and, more significantly, allowed no influence on adult personality or behaviour. The refusal of childhood (and with it, of course, the implicit refusal of the most radical development in understanding in the twentieth century which is psychoanalysis) is so striking a feature of auto/biography that it should – but seldom does – invite comment. Indeed, comment is scarcely sufficient to denote the misrepresentation that this facet of conventional auto/biography amounts to; it might be more appropriate to suggest that in this general refusal lies not just a problematic literary convention but a dominant cultural fault. Writing of two particularly disturbed patients, Marion Milner noted that both were deeply committed to a view of the world in which 'me' and 'not me' are sharply distinguished. She continued:

> But this (which is one possible meaning for the phrase 'premature ego development') leads them to great difficulties in managing their social environment, for they continually try to employ the kind of thinking (formal logic) which in fact gives a false picture of that world of human feeling (their own and other people's) that they are trying to understand and manage.[5]

The 'chaos within' to which all psychoanalysis at some point refers (and the management of which Milner discusses above) is, of course, a characteristic of human existence. We are all born with disordered and chaotic desires, which nevertheless are organised by the dominant infant needs for food and comfort. The material affluence of Europe in the twentieth century has made it possible for the material needs of infants to be satisfied in ways which are far more predictable than before, yet at the same time the spectre of the disorderly infant or child is still a haunting and problematic one for the culture of our prosperous societies. Infants are definitively not amenable to rational forms of social life, and their ability to achieve integration into society depends upon factors – most crucially, consistent mothering – which are in many ways marginal to societies that distance themselves from what is seen as 'nature'. Infants, and infancy, therefore remain a form of 'nature' which is general in any society, but different in kind to the rational expectations of the twentieth century. (The history of child and infant care in the twentieth century provides a particularly vivid example of this social tension about children. The early twentieth century saw considerable literature about 'training' children, by such figures as Truby King. After the Second World War, the era of Benjamin Spock and prominent child psychotherapists such as Anna Freud and Donald Winnicott was one in which the infant was to learn, and acquire, stability through stable relationships with others.[6])

Thus the time of infancy has a considerable sensitivity for apparently rational, bureaucratic societies. All societies desire citizens who are well integrated into their normative structure, but achieving that integration demands, it has become apparent, an acceptance of the disorder and chaos of infancy and childhood. The highly influential idea of infant feeding by a timetable introduced by Truby King is precisely representative of the wish of twentieth-century societies to dominate nature and literally to achieve mastery of natural desires. In the same way, auto/biographers in much of the twentieth century have refined the possibility of the emotional lives and motivations of their subjects, and fitted the life to the external expectations and the known realities. Thus, as a cultural and literary form, auto/

biography has had two remarkable features: first its almost complete and uncritical acceptance of social norms and conventions; and second its articulation of the social expectations about a person, rather than a discussion of the person her or himself.

Hence, therefore, the 'missing persons' of the title. The people who are missing from auto/biography are conventionally supposed to be the silent millions of people who have never achieved fame or notoriety, or even a place in recent oral or 'people's' history. Certainly, ordinary lives have until very recently had almost no appeal for auto/biographers and have been regarded as about as interesting as those years in history in which the grass grew. But the more truly 'missing' persons of auto/biography are not the silent millions but the subjects themselves, the people who have been subjected to the auto/biographer's gaze and still manage to remain rooted less in their own circumstances than the assumptions of the biographer. The refusal of childhood as a dominating experience in human experience in part accounts for this bias, but other factors that play their part include that intense twentieth-century hunger for the orderly control of existence, the form of the narrative of auto/biography and the facile twentieth-century assumption that information about sexual behaviour constitutes information about a 'private' life.

At the beginning of the twentieth century, the German sociologists Max Weber and Georg Simmel initiated definitive work on the psychological impact of Protestantism and capitalism. For Weber, the process of rationalisation in modern society led to both a loss of meaning in everyday life and an individual loss of control. He argued that:

> As intellectualism suppresses belief in magic, the world's processes become disenchanted, lose their magical significance, and henceforth simply 'are' and 'happen' but no longer signify anything. As a consequence, there is a growing demand that the world and the total pattern of life be subject to an order that is significant and meaningful.[7]

The last sentence stands as a particularly prescient comment on auto/biography: the 'growing demand' for order to which Weber refers fuels the inordinate desire of Western society in the twentieth century for coherent and systematic accounts of individual lives. Moreover, although many students of auto/biography have assumed that the genre has become more 'truthful' as standards and conventions about the explicit discussions of sexuality change, it can equally well be argued (and such is the argument here) that, although content may change (and become more or less superficially revelatory), the form stays the same, and it is a form with deep commitment to a given social order. Thus, contemporary auto/biography cannot in any sense 'reveal', because the author (and in equal measure the subject) has internalised the norms and conventions of the twentieth century. The search for the 'real' person is doomed to disappointment, for the two very good reasons that no 'real' person actually exists, and cannot be contained, let alone represented, in print. Nevertheless, the hope continues that somewhere, amidst more and more material, the 'real' person can be found.

But the prospect of 'real' people ever emerging from the pages of auto/biography is very limited. Part of the reason for this is that the very simplicities of our lives and our motivations are often obscured by the weight of auto/biographical information. In writing his fragment of auto/biography, Jean-Paul Sartre explicitly recognised the distinction between the meaning (to him) of his life and what could be said about him by others. Sartre's *Words* (uncharacteristically brief when compared with most of his other work) tells us everything we need to know about his motivation and his internal self.[8] We do not learn, as his subsequent biographers have told us, about his professional life or his relationships with other individuals, but we do know, from reading *Words*, that for this man access to and control of language was the be-all and end-all of existence. The context in which that passion was expressed remains, literally, a matter of record.

Yet despite the evidence that auto/biography itself provides, it is clear that the conventional view is that auto/biography is becoming in some sense more true to the person. The changed structures about revelation have fuelled an interpretation of twentieth-century auto/biography as emerging out of the dark night of repression, evasion and denial into a new dawn of frankness and openness. This reading of auto/biography takes little or no account of the way in which 'revelation' is a very movable feast, or the possibility that a discourse of, for example, the denial of the public discussion of sexuality is as revealing as any more open discussion. Those assumptions about the Victorian repression of an 'open' debate about sexuality are all derived from an understanding of cultural change which uncritically takes for granted a movement from the refusal to the acceptance of sexuality. Imbued with a sense of 'progress', in which the apparently more open discussion of sexuality is in some sense 'better' and 'enlightened', this view constructs its own emphases and biases which are, in their way, as misleading as those of the past. For example, in the bourgeois mores of Victorian England, strict codes governed the social circumstances in which individuals of the opposite sex could meet. We sometimes read this as a fear and refusal of sexuality, but we could equally read it as a recognition of the power of sexuality, and a recognition which had a crucial part to play in a society that rigidly organised personal morality.

To suppose, therefore, that auto/biography has, in some qualitative sense, 'improved' because it allows different material to be introduced, implies a tacit acceptance of twentieth-century assumptions about what constitutes 'modern' understanding. The 'modern' person, whether the auto/biographer or her or his subject, does not attempt to conceal her/his sexuality, let alone their relationships with others. The apparent excitements and turmoil of personal life can therefore take precedence over other events and situations in an individual's life – events as mundane, but as long-lasting and significant, as paid work and child-care. The impact of material need and constraint do not sit lightly with the assumptions of the late twentieth-century West; cultural shift has been such that it has been widely accepted that the individual can (and will) triumph, and that the difficulties we encounter in our lives are of our own making. In this discourse of individual responsibility it is all too easy to pathologise certain kinds of behaviour as inappropriate in terms of dominant discourses of 'healthy' or 'well-integrated' sexuality and/or personal behaviour.

The construction of the ideal self of the late twentieth century is one on which there is now a considerable and extensive literature. Body and mind have become the subject of discourses which assume a 'perfect' state of both appearance and function. The body appropriate to the late twentieth century is well-organised and well-ruled: it is a rational body and one which is not subject to 'unnecessary' diseases.[9] Living up to the body, rather than living in it or through it, has become a major industry which involves the control and organisation of nutrition, cosmetic surgery and the strict regulation of behaviour.[10] Equally, the ideal twentieth-century person is a person with the required functional skills for the labour market, a toleration of difference and diversity and an equally powerful ability to refuse 'extreme' ideas of any kind. This homogeneous person, in which differences of race or gender or class are increasingly regarded as irrelevant, is of course the perfect consumer and the perfect employee of late capitalism. It was the great ideological triumph of Thatcherism to convince large numbers of people that the 'natural' order of the world, indeed of human existence, was the market economy, and that the qualities of autonomy and independence are the pinnacles of human achievement.

Within a form of politics which has 'naturalised' capitalism, the function of auto/biography, and indeed its relationships to this context, is therefore one of allowing and organising the problematic human diversity of the real world. Biography was always a moralistic genre, in that biographers sought to demonstrate the moral worth or otherwise of their subjects, and provide estimation firmly rooted within early twentieth-century constructs of 'good' and 'bad' (and 'great' and 'evil'). The collapse of this discourse, which was firmly located within a rigid division

between the public and the private, shifted the ground for auto/
biographers away from the demonstration of moral qualities
towards the discussion and explanation of individual difference.
But in this shift the moral plurality of post-modernism came to
exercise considerable influence; individual people were no longer
to be assessed in terms of some kind of scale of moral achievement, they were to be seen as subjects of their own lives. Thus
arises the paradox of the late twentieth-century auto/biography:
as the culture becomes one of increasing conformity and pressures towards standardisation intensify, so auto/biography
becomes the literary articulation of difference. The more bizarre,
particularly in sexual terms, the subject can be made to appear,
the more attractive the auto/biography. Inevitably, the nature of
the 'bizarre' is all too often a construction. Given the variety
of human behaviour (and yet at the same time the similarity of
human need), it is inevitable that auto/biographers will construct
out of the same subject very different interpretations. These
interpretations have little to do with the 'truth' *per se*, but a great
deal to do with prevailing moral discourses and perceptions of
the acceptable extent of disclosure.

In the new climate of the auto/biography of revelation, it is
obviously important for some auto/biographers to maintain
their distance from those works which have achieved notoriety
through revelation. Thus, 'high' and 'low' auto/biography
regard each other with disdain and or contempt. Andrew Motion
on Philip Larkin is regarded as 'high' auto/biography, and
reviewers will speak of the work's contribution to auto/
biography and its place in the development of the genre. On the
other hand, Kitty Kelly on Frank Sinatra, Nancy Reagan or the
Windsors is regarded as beyond serious critical assessment. These
works all contain information which their subjects would clearly
prefer not to have discussed, and as such there is a case for
arguing that this is precisely the function of the auto/biographer
– to present the person that actually exists, rather than the person
of an individual's choice. However, this case is seldom put, and
the eighteenth-century model of Grub Street exposure is held up

as an invalid form of the practice of auto/biography. Motion, not Kelly, gets serious reviews and Kelly is used to illustrate, not the validity of the examination of the lives of the powerful, but the unacceptable and unscholarly in auto/biography. In this dichotomy we have to ask if auto/biography, a form which in many ways remains rooted in heroic narrative, does not further demonstrate its cultural lag. In the distinction between 'high' and 'low' auto/biography we find those aged arguments about high and low culture that have been a standard ingredient of the Anglo-Saxon literary world for decades. From the invention of Grub Street to Q.D. Leavis's *Fiction and the Reading Public* and T.S. Eliot's *Notes towards a Definition of Culture*, there has been a vocal (and influential) tradition within English literary criticism that has attempted to set itself apart from the profane world of mass culture.

In this dichotomy the 'sacred' auto/biography has been that which has accepted the definition of the subject as 'great' within a recognisable set of standards. Larkin stands as a major English poet, and what Motion does not do is to question what Larkin speaks for or about. The biography of Larkin was published in 1993, only eight years after Larkin's death. Yet as Hermione Lee points out in her biography of Virginia Woolf, Woolf had to wait years for any formal recognition by the same world that so rapidly embraced Larkin.[11] The contrast is important and telling, since Woolf was no outsider to English culture but a scion of the Establishment. Nevertheless, her gender and the nature of her work placed her on the margins of the culture for decades. It was only as the culture changed that Woolf became a subject to study. If the culture had not shifted in the way that it did (towards a much fuller recognition of the difference of women's writing and the articulation of a specifically female experience in modernity), it is likely that Woolf would still languish in obscurity.

Thus, as a guide to the past or the present, we must question the contribution of auto/biography. Shifts in cultural realms demand new figures; to suppose that in the study of auto/ biography we somehow regain a missing part of history or the present is to lose sight of the way in which we chose our subjects of auto/biography. Hence, the emphasis on the need for the uncovering of the working-class or female past leads to a focus on figures who, while interesting as all individuals are, may not in any sense represent anything more than individual interest. Yet the blurring of the boundary between the individual and the collective, which is a characteristic of post-modern culture, similarly informs auto/biography. Into the lives of diverse individuals we read cultural change and cultural phenomena. We cannot tolerate the ambiguity of human existence, and we thus provide ourselves with icons of experience and reality. In an age in which we assume that we can know and have access to all the secrets and motivations of existence, auto/biographers also insist on the struggle towards all-knowing information. The impossibility of this task suggests that we should view auto/biography as in urgent need of reclassification; that its place on the library shelves is not with non-fiction but very much closer to fiction. The 'real' person, whom the late twentieth century regards as a legitimate target for investigation, becomes less visible and less credible as we assume that all experience is individual rather than collective. The recognition of the shared frailty of human experience and human existence is largely out of step with the grandiose expectations of the late twentieth-century West. Since we cannot accept this collective experience, we are forced to construct ever more complex individuals to reassure ourselves of our individuality. In feeding the culture's desire for managed difference, auto/biography helps us to turn our backs on the shared circumstances of social life. As lives are not only lived in reality, so auto/biography provides us with the voyeuristic pleasures of experience.

Notes

1 The possibilities of auto/biography

1 See: Julia Kristeva, *Strangers to Ourselves* (New York, Columbia University Press, 1991).
2 Alfred P. Smyth, *King Alfred the Great* (Oxford, Oxford University Press, 1995), p. 149.
3 Michael Holroyd, *Lytton Strachey* (Harmondsworth, Penguin, 1971).
4 Roy Harrod, *The Life of John Maynard Keynes* (London, Macmillan, 1951).
5 The most famous such diary is that by George and Weedon Grossmith, *The Diary of a Nobody*, which describes the day-to-day life of a fictional London clerk, Charles Pooter. First published in 1892, it has been in print ever since.
6 Lytton Strachey, *Eminent Victorians* (London, Chatto and Windus, 1918).
7 For example, see the account of women's reactions to the First World War in Jan Montefiore, 'Shining Pins and Wailing Shells', in D. Goldman (ed.), *Women in World War I: The Written Response* (London, Macmillan, 1993), pp. 51–72.
8 Paul Fussell, *The Great War and Modern Memory* (Oxford, Oxford University Press, 1975).
9 See Siegfried Sassoon, *Memoirs of a Fox Hunting Man* (London, Faber and Faber, 1930) and Vera Brittain, *Testament of Youth* (London, Gollancz, 1933) and *Chronicle of Youth: Vera Brittain's War Diary 1913–1917* (London, Gollancz, 1981).
10 See Jan Montefiore, *Men and Women Writers of the 1930s* (London, Routledge, 1996).
11 George Orwell, *The Road to Wigan Pier* (London, Gollancz, 1936) and *Down and Out in Paris and London* (London, Gollancz, 1933).

12 Raphael Samuel, *Theatres of Memory* (London, Verso, 1994), p. 20.

13 Flora Thompson, *Lark Rise to Candleford* (Harmondsworth, Penguin, 1962).

14 Liz Stanley, *The Diaries of Hannah Cullwick* (London, Virago, 1984).

15 Liz Stanley, *The Auto/biographical I* (Manchester, Manchester University Press, 1992), p. 108.

16 Liz Stanley makes the point that Hannah Cullwick pre-empted later theoretical discussions in her implicit understanding of her position.

17 Liz Stanley, *The Auto/biographical I*, p. 108.

18 See, for example, the discussions in Doris Somner, 'Not just a Person Story: Women's Testimonies and the Plural Self', in B. Brodzki and Celeste Scherik (eds.), *Life/Lines: Theorising Women's Autobiography* (Ithaca, Cornell University Press, 1988), pp. 107–30.

19 Andrew Motion, *Philip Larkin: A Writer's Life* (London, Faber and Faber, 1993), p. 521.

20 Anne McClintock, *Imperial Leather: Race, Gender and Sexuality in the Colonial Contest* (London, Routledge, 1995).

21 See Leonard Woolf, *The Village in the Jungle* (London, 1913) and George Orwell, *Burmese Days* (London, Gollancz, 1929).

22 Max Weber, *The Protestant Ethic and the Spirit of Capitalism* (New York, Charles Scribner, 1958), p. 117.

23 Lucien Goldmann, *The Hidden God* (London, Routledge and Kegan Paul, 1964).

24 Lucien Goldmann, *The Hidden God*, p. 31.

25 The classic statement of this relationship is Ian Watt's *The Rise of the Novel* (Harmondsworth, Penguin, 1974).

26 Edward Said, *Culture and Imperialism* (London, Vintage Books, 1994), pp. 100–16.

27 Elaine Showalter, *Sexual Anarchy: Gender and Culture at the Fin de Siècle* (London, Virago, 1992), p. 60.

28 George Eliot, 'Silly Novels by Lady Novelists', *Westminster Review*, Vol. 4 (1856), pp. 442–61.

29 Michael Holroyd, Introduction to *Eminent Victorians* (London, Penguin, 1986), p. ix.

30 David Harvey, *The Condition of Post-Modernity* (Oxford, Blackwell, 1989), p. 19.

31 Lytton Strachey, *Eminent Victorians*, p. 160.

32 Alasdair Horne, Macmillan (London, Macmillan; Vol. I, 1988; Vol. II, 1989).

33 Judith R. Walkowitz, *Prostitution and Victorian Society: Women, Class and the State* (Cambridge, Cambridge University Press, 1983).

34 Sir Philip Magnus, *King Edward VII* (Harmondsworth, Penguin, 1972).

35 Philip Zeigler, *Mountbatten* (London, Fontana, 1986).
36 Jean-Paul Sartre, *Words* (Eng. trans. Harmondsworth, Penguin, 1967).

2 Lies, all lies: auto/biography as fiction

1 Simone de Beauvoir, *The Second Sex* (Eng. trans. New York, Bantam Books, 1964).
2 Simone de Beauvoir, *Les Belles Images* (Eng. trans. London, Fontana, 1977) and *The Woman Destroyed* (Eng. trans. London, Fontana, 1979).
3 Simone de Beauvoir, *Old Age* (Eng. trans. Harmondsworth, Penguin, 1978).
4 Nancy Armstrong, *Desire and Domestic Fiction: A Political History of the Novel* (Oxford, Oxford University Press, 1989).
5 See Jenny Uglow, *Elizabeth Gaskell* (London, Faber and Faber, 1995).
6 Toril Moi, *Simone de Beauvoir: The Making of an Intellectual Woman* (Oxford, Blackwell, 1994).
7 Kate Millett, *Sexual Politics* (London, Virago, 1977) and Shulamith Firestone, *The Dialectic of Sex* (New York, Bantam Books, 1971).
8 See Betty Friedan, *It Changed My Life: Writings on the Women's Movement* (New York, Random House, 1976).
9 Simone de Beauvoir, *Memoirs of a Dutiful Daughter* (Eng. trans. Harmondsworth, Penguin, 1963).
10 Simone de Beauvoir, *Memoirs of a Dutiful Daughter*, p. 136.
11 Simone de Beauvoir, *Memoirs of a Dutiful Daughter*, p. 141.
12 Simone de Beauvoir, *The Prime of Life* (Eng. trans. Harmondsworth, Penguin, 1965) and *Force of Circumstance* (Eng. trans. London, André Deutsch, 1965).
13 Simone de Beauvoir, *All Said and Done* (Eng. trans. Harmondsworth, Penguin, 1977).
14 Simone de Beauvoir, *All Said and Done*, p. 499.
15 Simone de Beauvoir, *All Said and Done*, p. 496.
16 Simone de Beauvoir, *The Prime of Life*, p. 22.
17 Deirdre Bair, *Simone de Beauvoir: A Biography* (London, Cape, 1990), pp. 514–16.
18 Simone de Beauvoir, *She Came to Stay* (Eng. trans. Harmondsworth, Penguin, 1966).
19 The real identity of 'M' is discussed by Deidre Bair in *Simone de Beauvoir*, p. 329.
20 Bianca Lamblin, *A Disgraceful Affair* Northeastern University Press, Mass., 1996).
21 Simone de Beauvoir, *The Prime of Life*, p. 528.

22 Simone de Beauvoir, *Force of Circumstance*, p. 10.
23 Nelson Algren, 'The Question of Simone de Beauvoir', *Harpers*, May 1965, pp. 134–6.
24 Simone de Beauvoir, *The Mandarins* (Eng. trans. London, Fontana, 1979).
25 Simone de Beauvoir, *The Mandarins*, p. 424.
26 Simone de Beauvoir, *A Very Easy Death* (Eng. trans. Harmondsworth, Penguin, 1969).
27 Simone de Beauvoir, *A Very Easy Death*, p. 89.
28 Janet Sayers, *Mothering Psychoanalysis*, (London, Hamish Hamilton, 1991), p. 230.
29 Simone de Beauvoir, *Memoirs of a Dutiful Daughter*, p. 289.
30 Deirdre Bair, *Simone de Beauvoir*, p. 459.
31 Deirdre Bair, *Simone de Beauvoir*, p. 459.
32 Deirdre Bair, *Simone de Beauvoir*, p. 459.
33 Deirdre Bair, *Simone de Beauvoir*, p. 11.
34 This position has been argued most forcefully by Sandra Harding in *Whose Science? Whose Knowledge?: Thinking from Women's Lives* (Milton Keynes, Open University Press, 1991).
35 For the relationship between Foucault and de Beauvoir, see David Macey, *The Lives of Michel Foucault* (London, Vintage, 1994), p. 446.

3 Imperatives of deference

1 Elizabeth Longford, *Victoria, R.I.* (London, Weidenfeld and Nicolson, 1964).
2 Elizabeth Longford, *Victoria, R.I.*, p. 649.
3 Kenneth Rose, *King George V* (London, Weidenfeld and Nicolson, 1983), p. 20.
4 Sir Philip Magnus, *King Edward VII* (Harmondsworth, Penguin, 1972).
5 Kenneth Rose, *King George V*, p. 53.
6 See Frances Donaldson, *Edward VIII* (London, Futura, 1974) and Philip Zeigler, *King Edward VIII* (London, Fontana, 1991).
7 Denis Judd, *King George VI* (London, Michael Joseph, 1982), p. 11.
8 Dorothy Thompson, *Queen Victoria: Gender and Power* (London, Virago, 1990), p. 41.
9 Kenneth Rose, *King George V*, p. 366.
10 Jonathan Dimbleby, *The Prince of Wales: A Biography* (London, Warner Books, 1995), pp. 68–94.
11 Philip Zeigler, *Edward VIII*, pp. 373–85.
12 Jonathan Dimbleby, *The Prince of Wales*, pp. 600–4.

13 Kenneth Rose, *King George V*, p. 215.
14 Kenneth Rose, *King George V*, p. 216.
15 Philip Zeigler, *Edward VIII*, p. 531.
16 See Stanley Weintrub, *Victoria: Biography of a Queen* (London, Unwin Hyman, 1987).
17 David Cannadine, *The Decline and Fall of the British Aristocracy* (London, Yale University Press, 1990).
18 Ben Pimlott, *The Queen* (London, HarperCollins, 1996).
19 Philip Zeigler, *Edward VII*, p. 559.
20 Ben Pimlott, *The Queen*; and Sarah Bradford, *Elizabeth: A Biography of Her Majesty the Queen* (London, Mandarin Books, 1997).

4 Boys' tales

1 See Ellen Moers, *Literary Women* (London, The Women's Press, 1978) and Sandra M. Gilbert and Susan Enbar, *The Madwoman in the Attic* (London, Yale University Press, 1984).
2 D.H. Lawrence, *Sons and Lovers* (Harmondsworth, Penguin, 1948).
3 David Morgan and Mary Evans, 'The Road to 1984', in Brian Brivati and Harriet Jones (eds.), *What Difference Did the War Make?* (London, Leicester University Press, 1993), pp. 37–48.
4 George Orwell, *A Clergyman's Daughter* (London, Gollancz, 1935) and *Keep the Aspidistra Flying* (London, Gollancz, 1936).
5 George Orwell, *The Road to Wigan Pier* (Harmondsworth, Penguin, 1966), p. 104.
6 George Orwell, *Down and Out in Paris and London* (Harmondsworth, Penguin, 1963), p. 99.
7 Michael Shelden, *Orwell* (New York, HarperCollins, 1991), p. 331.
8 George Orwell, 'Such, Such Were the Joys', *The Collected Essays, Journalism and Letters of George Orwell*, Vol. 4 (Harmondsworth, Penguin, 1970), pp. 379–423.
9 Michael Shelden, *Orwell*, p. 35.
10 See Janet Sayers, 'Sex Art and Reparation', *Women: A Cultural Review*, Vol. 1, No. 2, November 1990, pp. 135 44.
11 Gerald Brenan, *The Spanish Labyrinth* (London, Hamish Hamilton, 1943).
12 Evelyn Waugh, *A Little Learning* (London, Little Brown and Company, 1964).
13 Evelyn Waugh, *Brideshead Revisited* (Harmondsworth, Penguin, 1952), p. 27.
14 Evelyn Waugh, *Brideshead Revisited*, p. 79.
15 Evelyn Waugh, *Brideshead Revisited*, p. 168.
16 Z. Baumann, *Modernity and the Holocaust* (Cambridge, Polity, 1989).

17 David Lodge, *How Far Can You Go?* (Harmondsworth, Penguin, 1981), p. 58.
18 David Morgan and Mary Evans, *Battle For Britain* (London Routledge, 1993), p. 83.
19 Sylvia Plath, *The Bell Jar* (London, Faber and Faber, 1966).
20 Sylvia Plath, *The Bell Jar*, p. 85.
21 Sylvia Plath, *The Bell Jar*, p. 74.
22 See Pat Macpherson, *Reflecting on The Bell Jar* (London, Routledge, 1991).
23 Jacqueline Rose, *The Haunting of Sylvia Plath* (London, Virago, 1991).
24 This view is most vehemently argued by Sheila Jeffreys, *Anticlimax* (London, The Women's Press, 1990).
25 Maya Angelou, *I Know Why the Caged Bird Sings* (London, Virago, 1986).
26 Jeffrey Weeks, *Sexuality and its Discontents* (London, Routledge, 1985).
27 See the discussion in Edmund White, 'The Artist and AIDS', *Harper's Magazine*, 30 May 1987, pp. 22–3 and Oscar Moore, *Looking AIDS in the Face* (London, Picador, 1996).
28 Edmund White, *A Boy's Own Story* (London, Picador, 1983) and Geoffrey Wolff, *Duke of Deception* (New York, Vintage, 1990).
29 Angelica Garnett, *Deceived with Kindness: A Bloomsbury Childhood* (London, The Hogarth Press, 1984).
30 Angelica Garnett, *Deceived with Kindness*, p. 37.
31 John Osborne, *A Better Class of Person* (Harmondsworth, Penguin, 1988) and *Almost a Gentleman* (London, Faber and Faber, 1992).
32 John Osborne, *A Better Class of Person*, p. 37.
33 John Osborne, *A Better Class of Person*, p. 230.
34 Melanie Klein, *Envy and Gratitude and Other Works, 1946–1963* (London, The Hogarth Press, 1957).
35 John Osborne, *Almost a Gentleman*, p. 259.
36 Jane Austen, *Persuasion* (Harmondsworth, Penguin, 1965), p. 237.
37 George Orwell, *The Road to Wigan Pier*, p. 31.
38 Evelyn Waugh, *The Letters of Evelyn Waugh*, Mark Amory (ed.) (Harmondsworth, Penguin, 1982), p. 104.
39 Andrew Motion, *Philip Larkin: A Writer's Life* (London, Faber and Faber, 1994), p. 365.
40 Andrew Motion, *Philip Larkin*, p. 143.
41 Jan Morris, *Conundrum* (London, Faber and Faber, 1974).
42 Jan Morris, *Conundrum*, p. 158.
43 Jan Morris, *Conundrum*, p. 158.
44 Jan Morris, *Conundrum*, p. 138.
45 Jan Morris, *Conundrum*, p. 147.
46 Andrew Motion, *Philip Larkin*, p. xviii.

5 Looking for daddy

1 See Jan Montefiore, *Men and Women Writers of the 1930s* (London, Routledge, 1996).

2 See Marjorie Garber, *Vested Interests* (London, Penguin, 1993).

3 Elaine Showalter, *Sexual Anarchy: Gender and Culture at the Fin de Siècle* (London, Virago, 1992) and Sally Ledger, *The New Woman: Fiction and Feminism at the Fin de Siècle* (Manchester, Manchester University Press, 1997).

4 Elaine Showalter, *Sexual Anarchy*, p. 9.

5 Carol Gilligan, *In a Different Voice* (Cambridge, Mass., Harvard University Press, 1982).

6 Germaine Greer, *The Female Eunuch* (London, McGibbon and Kee, 1970) and *Sex and Destiny* (London).

7 Germaine Greer, *Daddy: We Hardly Knew You* (Harmondsworth, Penguin, 1990).

8 Germaine Greer, *Daddy, We Hardly Knew You*, p. 304.

9 Germaine Greer, *Daddy, We Hardly Knew You*, p. 21.

10 Germaine Greer, *Daddy, We Hardly Knew You*, p. 199.

11 Germaine Greer, *Daddy We Hardly Knew You*, p. 209.

12 Alice Kaplan, *French Lessons* (Chicago, University of Chicago Press, 1994), p. 209.

13 Alice Kaplan, *French Lessons*, p. 69.

14 Melanie Klein, 'Infantile anxiety situations reflected in a work of art and in the creative impulse', in Klein, *Love, Guilt and Reparation* (London, The Hogarth Press, 1975), p. 210.

15 Alice Kaplan, *French Lessons*, p. 69.

16 Sylvia Plath, *The Bell Jar*, p. 119.

17 Sylvia Plath, *The Bell Jar*, p. 88.

18 Betty Freidan, *The Feminine Mystique* (New York, Norton, 1963).

19 Carolyn Steedman, *Landscape for a Good Woman* (London, Virago, 1986), p. 39.

20 Valerie Walkerdine and Helen Lucey, *Democracy in the Kitchen: Regulating Mothers and Socialising Daughters* (London, Virago, 1989), p. 1.

21 This case is forcibly presented in Jacqueline Rose, *The Haunting of Sylvia Plath* (London, Virago, 1991).

22 Jacqueline Rose, *The Haunting of Sylvia Plath*, p. 232.

23 Janet Malcolm, *The Silent Woman: Sylvia Plath and Ted Hughes* (London, Picador, 1994).

24 Janet Malcolm, *The Silent Woman*, p. 177.

6 The imagined self: the impossibility of auto/biography

1 E.J. Hobsbawn, *Age of Extremes* (London, Michael Joseph, 1995) p. 543.
2 See Z. Baumann, *Modernity and the Holocaust* (Cambridge, Polity, 1989).
3 Martin Jay, *The Dialectical Imagination* (London, Heinemann, 1973).
4 Marion Milner, *The Suppressed Madness of Sane Men* (London, Tavistock, 1987).
5 Marion Milner, *The Suppressed Madness of Sane Men*, p. 232.
6 These disputes are discussed in Denise Riley, *War in the Nursery* (London, Virago, 1983).
7 Max Weber, quoted in David Frisby, *Fragments of Modernity* (Cambridge, Polity, 1985), p. 36.
8 Jean-Paul Sartre, *Words* (Eng. trans. Harmondsworth, Penguin, 1967).
9 Bryan Turner, *The Body and Society* (Oxford, Basil Blackwell, 1984).
10 Kathy Davis, *Re-Shaping the Female Body* (London, Routledge, 1995).
11 Hermione Lee, *Virginia Woolf* (London, Chatto and Windus, 1996), p. 13.

References

Algren, Nelson, May 1965. 'The Question of Simone de Beauvoir', *Harpers*, pp. 134–6.

Angelou, Maya, 1986. *I Know Why the Caged Bird Sings* (London, Virago).

Armstrong, Nancy, 1989. *Desire and Domestic Fiction: A Political History of the Novel* (Oxford, Oxford University Press).

Austen, Jane, 1965. *Persuasion* (Harmondsworth, Penguin).

Bair, Deidre, 1990. *Simone de Beauvoir: A Biography* (London, Cape).

Baumann, Z., 1989. *Modernity and the Holocaust* (Cambridge, Polity).

Beauvoir, Simone de, 1977. *All Said and Done* (Harmondsworth, Penguin).

Beauvoir, Simone de, 1969. *A Very Easy Death* (Harmondsworth, Penguin).

Beauvoir, Simone de, 1965. *Force of Circumstance* (London, André Deutsch).

Beauvoir, Simone de, 1977. *Les Belles Images* (London, Fontana).

Beauvoir, Simone de, 1963. *Memoirs of a Dutiful Daughter* (Harmondsworth, Penguin).

Beauvoir, Simone de, 1978. *Old Age* (Harmondsworth, Penguin).

Beauvoir, Simone de, 1966. *She Came to Stay* (Harmondsworth, Penguin).

Beauvoir, Simone de, 1979. *The Mandarins* (London, Fontana).

Beauvoir, Simone de, 1965. *The Prime of Life* (Harmondsworth, Penguin).

Beauvoir, Simone de, 1964. *The Second Sex* (New York, Bantam Books).

Beauvoir, Simone de, 1979. *The Woman Destroyed* (London, Fontana).

Brenan, Gerald, 1943. *The Spanish Labyrinth* (London, Hamish Hamilton).

Brittain, Vera, 1933. *Testament of Youth* (London, Gollancz).

Brittain, Vera, 1981. *Chronicle of Youth: Vera Brittain's War Diary 1913–1917* (London, Gollancz).

Cannadine, David, 1990. *The Decline and Fall of the British Aristocracy* (London, Yale University Press).

Davis, Kathy, 1995. *Re-Shaping the Female Body* (London, Routledge).

Dimbleby, Jonathan, 1995. *The Prince of Wales: A Biography* (London, Warner Books).

Donaldson, Frances, 1974. *Edward VIII* (London, Futura).

Eliot, George, 1856. 'Silly Novels by Lady Novelists', *Westminster Review*, Vol. 4, pp. 442–61.

Firestone, Shulamith, 1971. *The Dialectic of Sex* (New York, Bantam Books).

Freidan, Betty, 1963. *The Feminine Mystique* (New York, Norton).

Frisby, David, 1985. *Fragments of Modernity* (Cambridge, Polity).

Fussell, Paul, 1975. *The Great War and Modern Memory* (Oxford, Oxford University Press).

Garber, Marjorie, 1993. *Vested Interests* (London, Penguin).

Garnett, Angelica, 1984. *Deceived with Kindness: A Bloomsbury Childhood* (London, The Hogarth Press).

Gilbert, Sandra, M. and Enbar, Susan, 1984. *The Madwoman in the Attic* (London, Yale University Press).

Gilligan, Carol, 1982. *In a Different Voice* (Cambridge, Mass., Harvard University Press).

Greer, Germaine, 1970. *The Female Eunuch* (London, McGibbon and Kee).

Greer, Germaine, 1985. *Sex and Destiny* (London, Picador).

Greer, Germaine, 1990. *Daddy: We Hardly Knew You* (Harmondsworth, Penguin).

Goldmann, Lucien, 1964. *The Hidden God* (London, Routledge and Kegan Paul).

Harrod, Roy, 1951. *The Life of John Maynard Keynes* (London, Macmillan).

Harvey, David, 1989. *The Condition of Post-Modernity* (Oxford, Blackwell).

Hobsbawn, E.J. 1995. *Age of Extremes* (London, Michael Joseph).

Holroyd, Michael, 1971. *Lytton Strachey* (Harmondsworth, Penguin).

Holroyd, Michael, 1986. Introduction to Lytton Strachey, *Eminent Victorians* (London, Penguin).

Horne, Alasdair, 1988 and 1989. *Macmillan* (London, Macmillan, 2 vols).

Jay, Martin, 1973. *The Dialectical Imagination* (London, Heinemann).

Jeffreys, Sheila, 1990. *Anticlimax* (London, The Women's Press).

Judd, Denis, 1982. *King George VI* (London, Michael Joseph).

Kaplan, Alice, 1994. *French Lessons* (Chicago, University of Chicago Press).

Klein, Melanie, 1957. *Envy and Gratitude and Other Works, 1946–1963* (London, The Hogarth Press).

Klein, Melanie, 1975. *Love, Guilt and Reparation* (London, The Hogarth Press).

Kristeva, Julia, 1991. *Strangers to Ourselves* (New York, Columbia University Press).

Lamblin, Bianca, 1996. *A Disgraceful Affair* (Northeastern University Press, Mass.).

Lawrence, D.H., 1948. *Sons and Lovers* (Harmondsworth, Penguin).

Ledger, Sally, 1997. *The New Woman: Fiction and Feminism at the Fin de Siècle* (Manchester, Manchester University Press).

Lee, Hermione, 1996. *Virginia Woolf* (London, Chatto and Windus).

Lodge, David, 1981. *How Far Can You Go?* (Harmondsworth, Penguin).

Longford, Elizabeth, 1964. *Victoria, R.I.* (London, Weidenfeld and Nicolson).

Macey, David, 1993. *The Lives of Michel Foucault* (London, Vintage).

Magnus, Philip, 1972. *King Edward VII* (Harmondsworth, Penguin).

Malcolm, Janet, 1994. *The Silent Woman: Sylvia Plath and Ted Hughes* (London, Picador).

McClintock, Anne, 1995. *Imperial Leather: Race, Gender and Sexuality in the Colonial Contest* (London, Routledge).

Millet, Kate, 1977. *Sexual Politics* (London, Virago).

Milner, Marion, 1987. *The Suppressed Madness of Sane Men* (London, Tavistock).

Moers, Ellen, 1978. *Literary Women* (London, The Women's Press).

Moi, Toril, 1994. *Simone de Beauvoir: The Making of an Intellectual Woman* (Oxford, Blackwell).

Montefiore, Jan, 1993. 'Shining Pins and Wailing Shells', in Goldman, D. (ed.) *Women in World War I: The Written Response* (London, Macmillan).

Montefiore, Jan, 1996. *Men and Women Writers of the 1930s* (London, Routledge).

Morgan, David and Evans, Mary, 1993. *Battle for Britain* (London, Routledge).

Morgan, David and Evans, Mary, 1993. 'The Road to 1984' in

Brivati, B. and Jones, Harriet (eds.) *What Difference did the War Make?* (London, Leicester University Press).

Morris, Jan, 1974. *Conundrum* (London, Faber and Faber).

Motion, Andrew, 1993. *Philip Larkin: A Writer's Life* (London, Faber and Faber).

Orwell, George, 1929. *Burmese Days* (London, Gollancz).

Orwell, George, 1933. *Down and Out in Paris and London* (London, Gollancz).

Orwell, George, 1935. *A Clergyman's Daughter* (London, Gollancz).

Orwell, George, 1936. *The Road to Wigan Pier* (London, Gallancz).

Orwell, George, 1936. *Keep the Aspidistra Flying* (London, Gollancz).

Orwell, George, 1970. *The Collected Essays, Journalism and Letters of George Orwell*, Vol. 4 (Harmondsworth, Penguin).

Osborne, John, 1988. *A Better Class of Person* (Harmondsworth, Penguin).

Osborne, John, 1992. *Almost a Gentleman* (London, Faber and Faber).

Pimlott, Ben, 1996. *The Queen* (London, HarperCollins).

Plath, Sylvia, 1966. *The Bell Jar* (London, Faber and Faber).

Riley, Denise, 1983. *War in the Nursery* (London, Virago).

Rose, Jacqueline, 1991. *The Haunting of Sylvia Plath* (London, Virago).

Rose, Kenneth, 1983. *King George V* (London, Weidenfeld and Nicolson).

Said, Edward, 1994. *Culture and Imperialism* (London, Vintage Books).

Samuel, Raphael, 1994. *Theatres of Memory* (London, Verso).

Sartre, Jean-Paul, 1967. *Words* (Harmondsworth, Penguin).

Sassoon, Siegfried, 1930. *Memoirs of a Fox Hunting Man* (London, Faber).

Sayers, Janet, 1990. 'Sex, Art and Reparation', *Women: A Cultural Review*, Vol. 1, No. 2.

Sayers, Janet, 1991. *Mothering Psychoanalysis* (London, Hamish Hamilton).

Shelden, Michael, 1991. *Orwell* (New York, HarperCollins).

Showalter, Elaine, 1992. *Sexual Anarchy: Gender and Culture at the Fin de Siècle* (London, Virago).

Smyth, Alfred, P. (1995). *King Alfred the Great* (Oxford, Oxford University Press).

Somner, Doris, 1988. 'Not just a Person Story: Women's Testimonies and the Plural Self", in Brodzki, B. and Scherik, C. (eds), *Life/Lines: Theorising Women's Autobiography* (Ithaca, Cornell University Press).

Stanley, Liz, 1984. *The Diaries of Hannah Cullwick* (London, Virago).

Stanley, Liz, 1992. *The Auto/biographical I* (Manchester, Manchester University Press).

Steedman, Carolyn, 1986. *Landscape for a Good Woman* (London, Virago).

Strachey, Lytton, 1918. *Eminent Victorians* (London, Chatto and Windus).

Thompson, Dorothy, 1990. *Queen Victoria: Gender and Power* (London, Virago).

Turner, Bryan, 1984. *The Body and the Society* (Oxford, Basil Blackwell).

Uglow, Jenny, 1995. *Elizabeth Gaskell* (London, Faber and Faber).

Walkerdine, Valerie and Lucey, Helen, 1989. *Democracy in the Kitchen: Regulating Mothers and Socialising Daughters* (London, Virago).

Walkowitz, Judith, R. 1983. *Prostitution and Victorian Society: Women, Class and the State* (Cambridge, Cambridge University Press).

Waugh, Evelyn, 1952. *Brideshead Revisited* (Harmondsworth, Penguin).

Waugh, Evelyn, 1964. *A Little Learning* (London, Little Brown and Company).

Waugh, Evelyn, 1982. *The Letters of Evelyn Waugh*, ed. Mark Amory (Harmondsworth, Penguin).

Weber, Max, 1958. *The Protestant Ethic and the Spirit of Capitalism* (New York, Charles Scribner).

Weeks, Jeffrey, 1985. *Sexuality and its Discontents* (London, Routledge).

Weintrub, Stanley, 1987. *Victoria: Biography of a Queen* (London, Unwin Hyman).

White, Edmund, 1983. *A Boy's Own Story* (London, Picador).

White, Edmund, 1987. 'The Artist and AIDS', *Harper's Magazine*, 30 May, pp. 22–3.

Woolf, Leonard, 1913. *The Village in the Jungle* (London).

Zeigler, Philip, 1986. *Mountbatten* (London, Fontana).

Zeigler, Philip, 1991. *King Edward VIII* (London, Fontana).

Index